Grigori Grabovoi

Restoration of Matter of Human Being by

Concentrating on Number Sequence

The work „Restoration of Matter of Human Being by
Concentrating on Number Sequence" was created and supplemented
by Grigori Grabovoi in 2002.

Hamburg

2012

Jelezky Publishing, Hamburg

www.jelezky-publishing.com

First English Edition, October 2012

© 2012 English Language Edition

SVET UG, Hamburg (Publisher)

Published by SVET UG, Hamburg, Germany 2012

Cover Design: Sergey Jelezky, www.jelezky.com

For further information on the contents of this book contact:

SVET Centre, Hamburg

www.svet-centre.com

ISBN: 978-3-943110-54-8

According to the responses we have received, the contents of this book have helped many people. We are confident that this will continue to be the case.

Nonetheless, we would like to point out that the techniques of Grigori Grabovoi are mental methods for the guidance of events in one's life. These methods are dependent upon one's personal spiritual development. Because we are dealing with topics relating to one's health, we give this express notice that such influence is not a "therapy" in the conventional sense of the word and is therefore not intended to limit or replace professional medical care.

When in doubt, follow the directions of your doctor or a therapist or pharmacist whom you trust!

(When following conventional methods, you must expect to get conventional results.)

Jelelezky Publishing/SVET Centre, Hamburg

Disclaimer:

The information within this book is intended as reference material only, and not as medical or professional advice.

Information contained herein is intended to give you the tools to make informed decisions about your lifestyle. It should not be used as a substitute for any treatment that has been prescribed or recommended by your qualified doctor. Do not stop taking any medication unless advised by your qualified doctor to do otherwise. The author and publisher are not healthcare professionals, and expressly disclaim any responsibility for any adverse effects occurring as a result of the use of suggestions or information in this book. This book is offered for your own education and enjoyment only. As always, never begin a health program without first consulting a qualified healthcare professional. Your use of this book indicates your agreement to these terms.

INTRODUCTION

To restore the matter of human being with the numerical concentrations the following methods can be used:

1. Read the number sequence corresponding to matter being restored, written after the name of matter.

2. Pronounce mentally the number sequence corresponding to the matter being restored.

3. Look at the picture or the name of the matter being restored.

4. Imagine that you are situated between the numbers of the sequence, having big size, corresponding to the matter being recreated. You must strive to perceive clearly the numbers, between which you imagine yourself. The light of these numbers can reach you. These actions can be performed with any numbers of sequence.

5. Imagine that you are looking at the number sequence from above.

6. Imagine the number sequence in that area which you are restoring. To do this, you must use the image of the matter, given in this book, with the sequence of numbers you are using.

7. Imagine the number sequence between the picture of the matter and a

4 \qquad © Г.П. Грабовой 2002

part of the specular reflection, given in this book, which correspond to the number sequence being used.

8.   Comparing the numbers of the sequence, you can find a controlling relationship between the various kinds of human matter in the direction to norm. It is possible to restore the matter, using the number sequence corresponding to the other matter. At first you can concentrate on the numbers of the sequence of the other matter, which coincide with the numbers of the sequence of the matter being restored. Then you can use the whole sequence of numbers of the other matter, drawing in your thoughts a light beam which crosses the number sequence of the matter or the matter itself which you are restoring. At the perception of the rapid restoring effect you can define the next point or area in your body after the restored matter itself, through which the matter is recreated. This next point or area in such a case will be situated in the other matter, with the help of the number sequence of which the restoration of the matter, chosen by you, is carried out. There could be a lot of such following points or areas through which the creation of the matter is performed. The first point or area of the selected matter is in the matter itself.

Having found, through the use of number sequence, the points or areas of creation of the matter being restored, one can recreate the matter focusing his attention on these points or areas. At this time such a spiritual state sets in that corresponds to the restoration and the normal state of the chosen matter. Bringing back to memory and feeling again the same spiritual state, you can restore the matter by means of spirit, which thus is a Life-giving Spirit. Then you can extend this spiritual act to the whole matter of the body taking into account external events and thus achieve a spiritual state, corresponding to the eternal development.

In certain cases, depending on the angle of perception, different number sequences can correspond to the same matter being restored.

9.   To accelerate the restoration of the human matter the gaps in the number sequences can be perceived as the gaps between the words in a sentence. Then for each component of a number sequence, separated by the gap, one can see a word that has a meaning of a normally functioning matter to which given number sequence corresponds. Then, trying to perceive this word, it is possible to perceive the Creator's level creating the matter that corresponds to the number sequence and the matter of the whole body. Light, creating the matter corresponding to the number sequence, is spread, according to the laws of optics, to all other matters of the human body and to the environment. From this you can understand why some feelings and emotions are perceived as external. This allows to recognize more accurately where on the level of control over events it is necessary to act on the basis of the interaction of body tissues and where on the basis of the interaction of the matter of the organism and the environment. This method of the exact detection allows you to make control over events more efficiently until the level of the normal state of matter of the body is reached, regardless of any circumstances.

With this method you perceive simultaneously both tissue of the body and the events surrounding a man in such a way as though you are looking at the described above with the physical eyes. And depending on situation, you can make a decision how to act in the direction of eternal development. In some cases you can perform physical actions, and in some periods you can perform a spiritual action for the normalization of the events in the direction to the eternal life.

Such perception of yours develops your spirit, soul and physical body to the level at which the creation of human matter is fulfilled on spiritual basis. Figures make it possible to get the exact spiritual state, corresponding to the norm of human matter. To strengthen the control you can use common known, that is well fixed in the collective consciousness, knowledge from physics, about the corpuscular-wave duality of matter, according to which any object can show both its wave properties and particle characteristics of matter. Creating the light waves by concentration on the number sequence corresponding to the normal human matter, you create normally functioning human matter.

All the methods of restoration of human matter with the help of concentration on number sequences given in this book can be used with preventive and sanitary purposes, for rejuvenation, and in case of necessity, to restore the matter, regardless of the initial data, on the basis of which the matter is restored. When using the described methods in paragraphs 1-9 in the introduction you can consider the following:

With the aim of prophylaxis it is expedient to make rehabilitation with the simultaneous spreading the effect of concentration on number sequences for the future.

For rejuvenation it is expedient to concentrate in succession at first on the number sequence, located in the content (of the book), taking into account the task of eternal development, and then concentrate on the matter which you are locally rejuvenating.

Restoring the matter of the body, you can perform concentration on number sequences in succession with the help of the various methods given in this book. You can use the number sequences corresponding to the matter being restored, as well as the number sequences of the area, which includes the matter you are restoring.

If it is necessary to restore the matter after biological death, then you should at first concentrate on the numbers consecutively from left to right, then in reverse order – from right to left.

The spiritual impulse creating human matter makes it possible to expand the methods of restoration. Restoring the human matter one must strive to develop the spiritual level to the state in which the matter is created and functions by the spiritual activity, along with the biological principles and principles of events. Such spiritual state in the process of implementation of the methods of the eternal development must ensure full restoration of human matter, regardless of the initial data and any circumstances.

CELLS AND TISSUES 829 3791 429 841 *

* In the first edition of this book 13- figures number sequence is included as well as some other methods in order to strengthen stability of control in case of inattentiveness of a user. The aim of these methods is to have such concentration that stays stable even if the user by mistake says mentally another figure.

CELLS 319 078 121 942

Fig. 1. Cells Forms:

1 — nerve cell (neuron) 519 513 819 814

2 — epithelial cell 518 321 678 024

3 — connective tissue cell 819 417 319 814

4 — smooth muscle cell 519 312 419 814

5 — erythrocyte 214 719 319 818

6 — sperm cell 319 814 888 918

7 — egg (ovule) 888 319 914 718

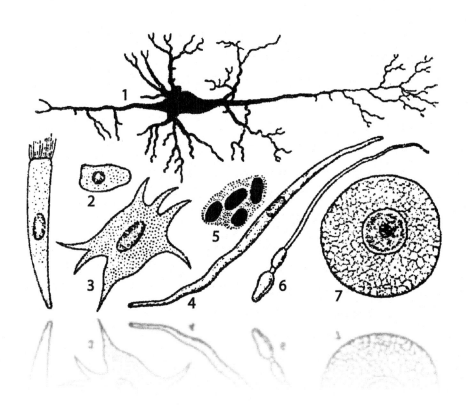

Fig. 2. Ultramicroscopic Cell Structure:

1 — cytolemma (plasma membrane) 814 718 314 213

2 — pinocytie vesicles 214 718 314 218

3 — centrosome (cell center, cytocentrum) 519 217 018 017

4 — hyaloplasm 614 217 321 218

5 — endoplasmic reticulum 819 517 319 418

(a — membranes of the endoplasmic reticulum,

b — ribosomes)

6 — cell nucleus 814 321 718 912

7 — centact of perinuclear space with cavities of the endoplasmic
    reticulum 819 421 719 378

8 — nuclear pores 918 472 519 318

9 — endosome (cell nucleolus) 918 412 718 814

10 — net intracellular apparatus (Golgi complex) 819 918 319 217

11 — secretory vacuoles 979 974 348 522

12 — mitochondria 819 317 419 814

13 — lysosomes 519 712 314 518

14 — three suceessive stages of phagocytosis 819 412 714 321

15 — connection of cell membrane with membranes of endoplasmic
    reticulum 514 816 314 819

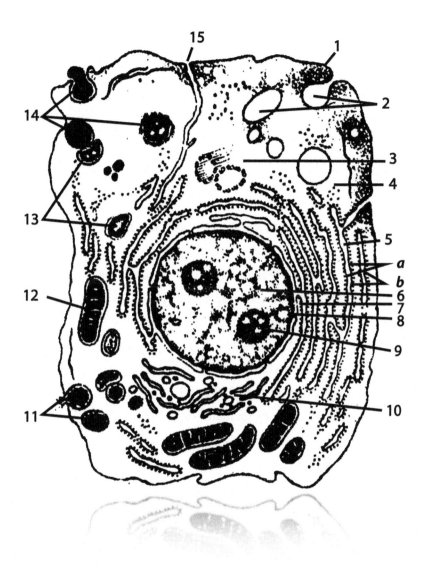

TISSUE 898 314 988 889

EPITHELIAL TISSUE 891 389 426 319

Fig. 3. Various types of epithelium:

A — single – layered squamous epithelium 819 417 319 817

B — single – layered cuboidal epithelium 514 312 814 712

C — cylindrical epithelium 318 216 718 916

D — ciliated epithelium 319 821 319 719

E — pseudostratified epithelium 918 216 917 418

F — stratified keratinizing epithelium 418 217 218 317

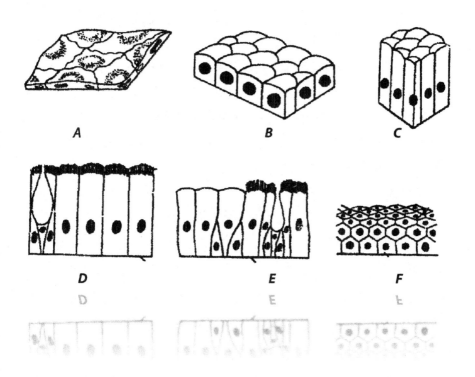

A   B   C

D   E   F

CONNECTIVE TISSUE 719 317 918 517

MUSCLE TISSUE 514 312 814 312

Fig. 4. Types of muscle Tissue:

I — longitudinal view

II — cross-section view

A — smooth muscle 514 718 314 218

B — striated skeletal muscle 917 312 218 412

C — striated cardiac muscle 914 318 514 712

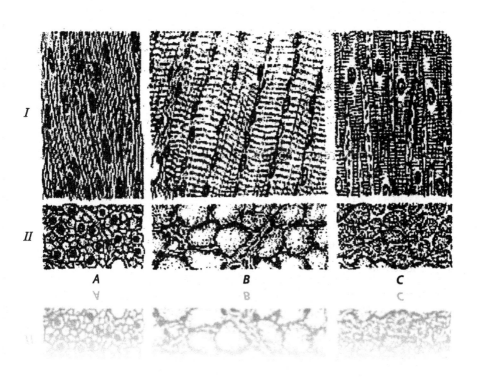

I

II

A   B   C

19

NERVOUS TISSUE 718 412 518 914

Fig. 5. Structure of neuron:

I — sensory neuron 814 317 914 918:

1 — nerve endings 519 312 214 712

2 — axon 314 812 219 418

3 — nucleus of neuron 314 812 219 217

4 — cell body 917 219 817 519

5 — dendrite 318 517 918 241

6 — myelin sheath 514 717 814 317

7 — receptor 518 214 019 481

8 — organ 814 317 914 817

9 — nevrilemma 714 312 814 512

II — motor neuron 319 816 819 312:

1 — dendrites 519 321 819 428

2 — axon 419 218 519 321

3 — terminal plaque 214 217 814 312

4 — nodes of Ranvier 518 217 818 217

5 — Schwann cell nucleus 214 312 814 212

6 — Schwann cell 841 218 412 518

III — Intercalated neuron 314 517 214 817:

1 — axon 314 812 219 418

2 — dendrites 317 518 919 318

3 — nucleus 489 218 219 311

4 — cell body 518 218 918 317

5 — dendrite 518 418 719 281

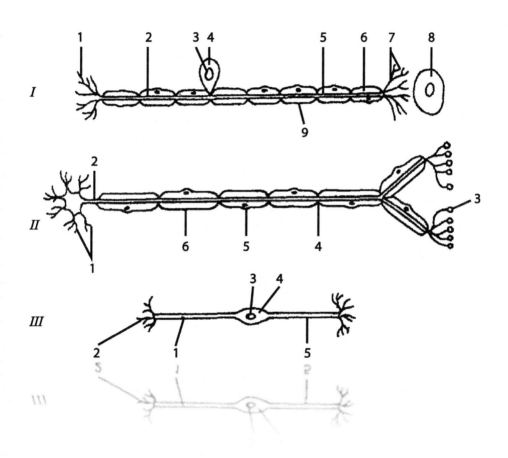

Fig. 6. Types of neurons:

A — unipolar neuron 514 312 814 212

B — diaxon 818 217 318 514

C — multipolar neuron 514 712 814 312

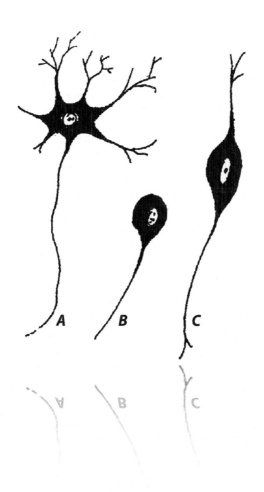

A   B   C

NERVOUS SYSTEM 219 317 819 298

CENTRAL NERVOUS SYSTEM 291 384 074 217

SPINAL CORD 314 218 814 719

Fig. 7. Spinal cord (diagram):

A: 1 — Spinal cord 219 381 478 064

2 — cervical intumescence 298 387 984 721

3 — lumbo – sacral intumescence 429 317 219 817

4 — medullary cone 219 381 419 971

5 — terminal filum 519 317 919 218

B: 1 — terminal ventricle 419 814 218 914

2 — terminal filum 519 312 819 212

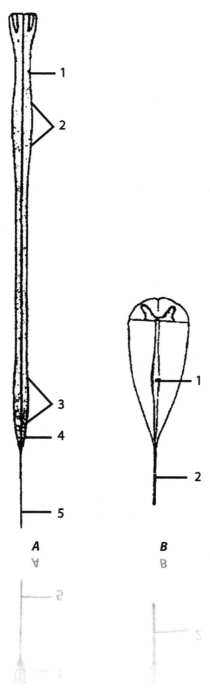

A

B

Fig. 8. Segments of spinal cord 219 317 888 847:

1 — cervical segments (1 — 8) 218 828 204 217,

      cervical part 849 218 314 918

2 — thoracic segments (1 — 12), thoracic part 234 891 019 217

3 — lumbar segments (1 — 5), lumbar part 219 004 489 668

4 — sacral segments (1 — 5), sacral part 229 317 916 021

5 — coccygeal segments (1 — 3), coccygeal part 834 219 918 715

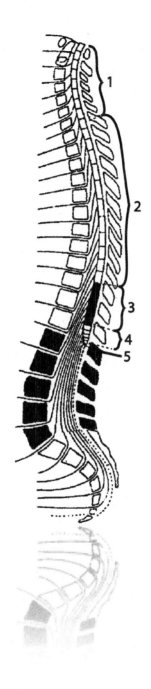

Fig. 9. Spinal cord (diagram):

1 — central canal 888 991 213 451

2 — gray matter 891 021 328 423

3 — white matter 478 217 219 328

4 — anterior funiculus 489 219 219 321

5 — lateral funiculus 290 029 432 517

6 — posterior funiculus 048 217 428 471

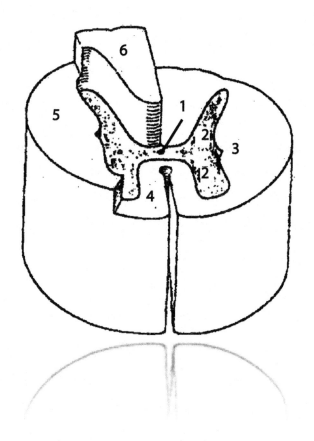

Fig. 10. Columns of gray matter in spinal cord:

1 — posterior 219 482 319 213

2 — lateral 214 712 218 521

3 — anterior 317 484 217 244

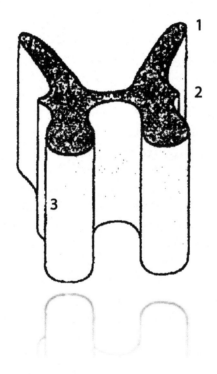

Fig. 11. Conductive pathways of white
matter (cross- section of spinal cord) (scheme):

1 — gracile fasciculus 219 317 418 217

2 — cuneate fasciculus 319 215 219 317

3 — posterior root of spinal nerve 214 317 219 224

4 — lateral cortico-spinal (pyramidal) tract 248 317 218 321

5 — rubro nuclear spinal tract 428 521 328 721

6 — posterior spinal cerebellar tract 888 917 218 912

7 — anterior spinal cerebellar tract 918 214 218 217

8 — lateral spinal thalamic tract 318 217 218 914

9 — spino-olivary tract 514 219 314 819

10 — vestibulo spinal tract 219 444 558 913

11 — reticulo spinal tract 219 317 418 213

12 — anterior cortico-spinal (pyramidal) tract 219 318 214 217

13 — anterior spinal – thalamic tract 219 317 218 214

14 — tecto spinal tract 218 317 219 217

15 — posterior, lateral and anterior own fasciculus 219 314 214 315

16 — anterior horn 218 217 314 218

17 — lateral horn 218 317 214 218

18 — posterior horn 418 217 218 317

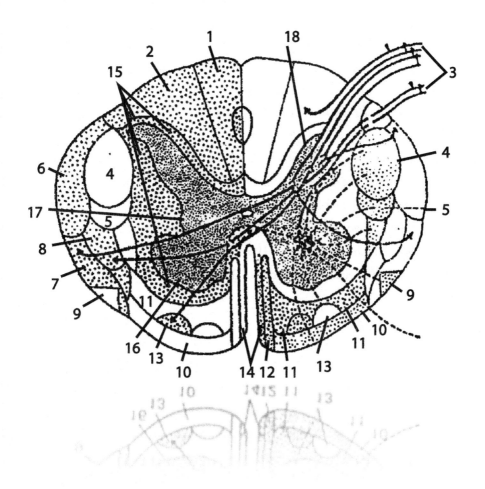

Fig. 12. Spinal cord membranes 219 317 819 312:

1 — spinal pia mater 849 312 219 814

2 — subarachnoid space 314 712 814 212

3 — spinal arachnoid mater 219 317 814 218

4 — spinal dura mater 218 217 319 218

5 — epidural space 217 314 218 217

6 — dentate ligament 217 318 219 312

7 — intermedial cervical septum 214 321 814 712

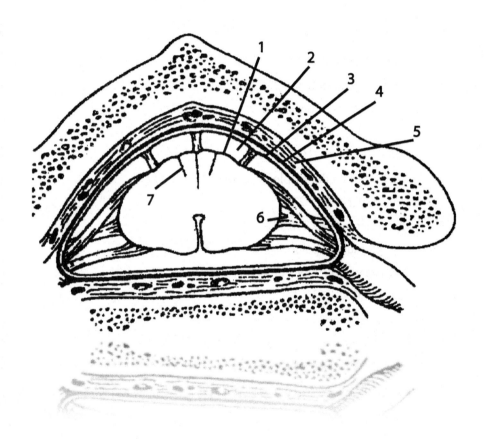

BRAIN 814 729 318 818

Fig. 13. Base of brain 219 888 676 021:

1 — olfactory analyser bulb 024 312 598 742

2 — olfactory tract 718 217 458 917

3 — anterior perforated substance 218 317 219 218

4 — tuber cinereum 519 317 219 417

5 — optic tract 519 218 919 245

6 — mammillary bodies 534 817 214 712

7 — trigeminal ganglion 418 217 218 217

8 — posterior perforated substance 219 317 919 217

9 — pons 248 317 284 271

10 — cerebellum 828 219 328 299

11 — pyramid of medulla oblongata 928 321 728 521

12 — olive 489 217 319 271

13 — spinal nerves 489 218 918 217

14 — hypoglossus (hypoglossal nerve) 548 321 555 678

15 — accessory nerve 489 917 319 712

16 — vagus 489 981 728 221

17 — glossopharyngeal nerve 519 371 214 572

18 — vestibulocochlear nerve 548 217 918 421

19 — facialis 999 811 319 211

20 — abducens 514 517 214 812

21 — trigeminal nerve 519 312 819 212

22 — trochlear nerve 319 712 819 212

23 — motor oculi 519 217 519 217

24 — optic nerve 448 817 918 217

25 — olfactory nerves 478 215 589 315

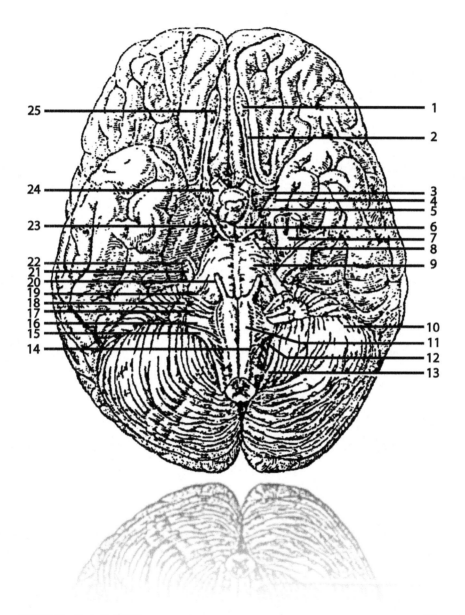

25 ——————————————————— 1

2

24 ——————————————————— 3
4
5
23 ——————————————————— 6
7
8
22 ——————————————————— 9
21
20
19
18
17
16 ——————————————————— 10
15 ——————————————————— 11
14 ——————————————————— 12
13

Fig. 14. Brain (sagittal view):

1 — sulcus of the corpus callosum 248 312 848 212

2 — cingulate sulcus 579 312 919 021

3 — cingulate gyrus 898 312 024 712

4 — callosum 498 712 328 071

5 — central sulcus 489 213 048 217

6 — paracentral lobule 811 017 319 218

7 — calcarine sulcus 214 318 414 888

8 — quadrigeminal plate 514 317 818 212

9 — cerebellum 828 219 328 299

10 — fourth ventricle 514 321 414 218

11 — medulla oblongata 514 417 814 217

12 — pons 519 312 819 212

13 — pineal body (epiphysis) 519 317 819 217

14 — cerebral peduncles 918 412 818 212

15 — pituitary gland 317 218 219 819

16 — third ventricle 818 217 418 217

17 — interthalamic symphysis 819 312 919 222

18 — pellucid septum 214 817 914 817

19 — superior frontal gyrus 918 918 919 217

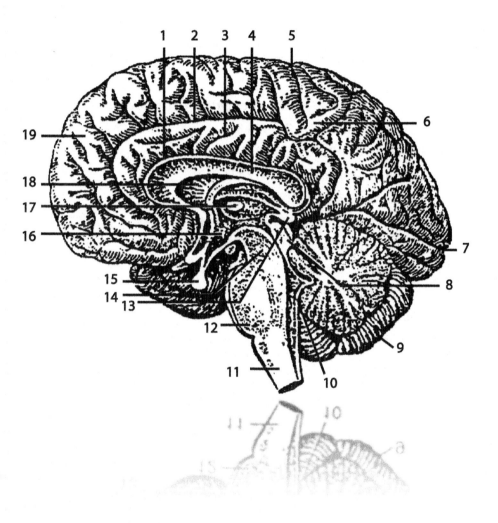

MEDULLA OBLONGATA (MYELENCEPHALON) 214 713 914 819

Fig. 15. Medulla oblongata (ventral view):

1 — medulla oblongata 214 713 914 819

2 — retro olive area 219 317 919 817

3 — anterior median fissure 914 712 814 212

4 — retro olive sulcus 319 217 819 317

5, 9 — anterior lateral sulcus 519 310 819 210

6 — anterior external arcuate fibers 918 217 918 719

7 — pyramidal decussation 910 918 819 312

8 — lateral funiculus 314 912 814 712

10 — olive 514 312 814 912

11 — pyramid of medulla oblongata 519 317 919 817

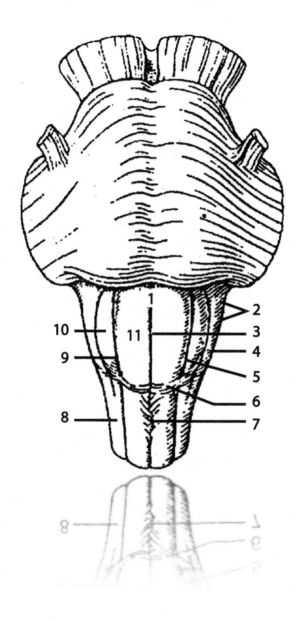

43

HINDBRAIN 219 317 219 817
PONS AND CEREBELLUM 219 317 919 217

Fig. 16. Hindbrain (Metencephalon) 219 317 219 817:

1 — cerebellum 828 219 328 299

2 — cerebellopontine triangle (pontocerebellar trigone) 214 312 814 912

3 — bulbopontine sulcus 819 312 219 217

4 — basilar sulcus 519 312 219 212

5 — middle cerebellar peduncle 219 710 819 210

6 — pons 519 312 219 224

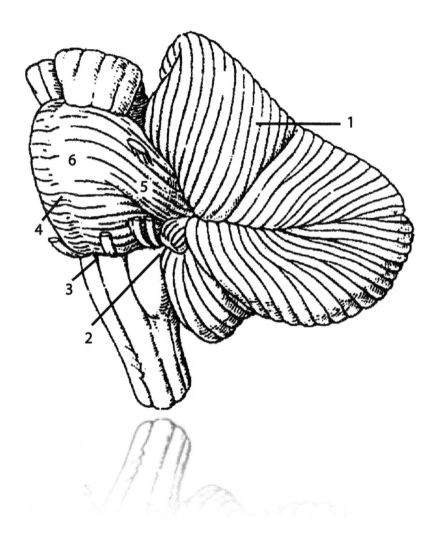

Fig. 17. Transverse View of Pons (diagram):

1 — posterior longitudinal fasciculus 519 317 819 213

2 — midbrain tract of trigeminal nerve 519 017 819 317

3 — medial longitudinal fasciculus 517 918 917 819

4 — medial loop (lemniscus) 319 021 713 211

5 — reticular formation 519 312 919 812

6 — trigeminal loop (lemniscus) (trigeminal-thalamic tract) 819 417 919 817

7 — spinal lemniscus 514 312 914 212

8 — cerebellopotine fibers 519 471 919 012

9 — corticonuclear fibers 519 315 219 818

10 — cortico-pontine fibers 519 317 919 817

11 — pontine nuclei 514 312 914 214

12 — cortico-spinal fibers 218 319 219 418

13 — basilar sulcus 519 318 914 218

14 — transverse pontine fibers 519 312 919 218

15 — anterior (basilar) part of pons 588 217 918 214

16 — posterior part of pons (pons tegmentum) 819 312 919 212

17 — raphe of pons 519 318 919 218

18 — tectospinal tract 518 217 918 217

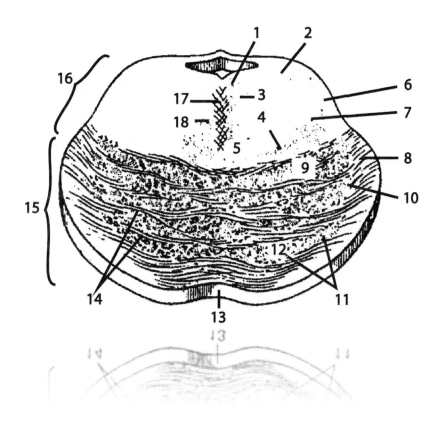

MIDBRAIN (MESENCEPHALON) 519 417 819 210

Fig. 18. Midbrain and rhomboid fossa 519 317 888 910:

1 — cover plate (of quadrigemina) 519 817 319 217

2 — superior cerebellar peduncle 419 817 919 217

3 — loop triangle 519 217 314 717

4 — lower colliculus 514 817 914 917

5 — upper colliculus 918 071 518 971

6 — brachium of inferior colliculus 519 217 918 201

7 — brachium of superior colliculus 519 322 068 290

DIENCEPHALON 919 213 819 223

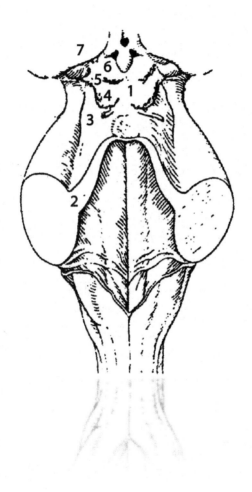

Fig. 19. Brain: upper lateral surface,
furrows and convolutions (sulci and gyri) (diagram):

A, B: 1 — lateral sulcus 514 213 814 213

2 — tegmental (opercular) part of inferior frontal gyrus 219 312 819 222

3 — triangular part of inferior frontal gyrus 888 917 918 217

4 — orbital part of inferior frontal gyrus 519 312 219 212

5 — inferior frontal sulcus 498 213 718 223

6 — inferior frontal gyrus 519 312 519 212

7 — superior frontal sulcus 514 317 514 817

8 — middle frontal gyrus 514 017 314 917

9 — superior frontal gyrus 918 217 518 917

10 — inferior precentral sulcus 519 217 919 817

11 — superior precentral sulcus 918 512 318 412

12 — precentral gyrus 479 318 012 891

13 — central sulcus 999 613 918 213

14 — postcentral sulcus 519 217 918 227

15 — intraparietal sulcus 418 218 219 371

16 — superior parietal lobule 514 318 914 818

17 — inferior parietal lobule 514 319 214 819

18 — supramarginal gyrus 918 883 518 913

19 — angular gyrus 519 311 918 911

20 — occipital pole 519 317 819 517

21 — inferior temporal sulcus 519 217 219 317

22 — superior temporal gyrus 519 218 919 519

23 — middle temporal gyrus 519 712 919 212

24 — inferior temporal gyrus 518 317 918 217

25 — superior temporal sulcus 514 219 314 919

50

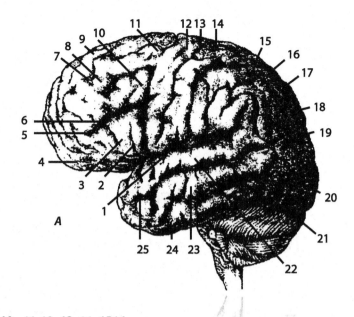

A

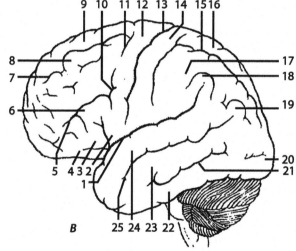

B

BRAIN VENTRICLES 219 317 919 217

Fig. 20. Lateral ventricles of cerebrum 919 814 919 217:

1 — central part of lateral ventricle 514 312 814 712

2 — inferior horn 319 817 919 917

3 — posterior horn 519 317 919 817

4 — interventricular foramen 548 321 918 811

5 — septum pellucidum 519 317 819 217

6 — head of caudate nucleus 511 064 918 244

7 — anterior horn 514 312 518 212

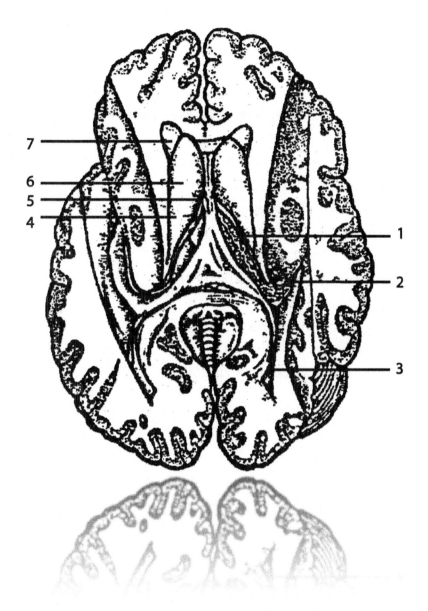

Fig. 21. Rhombencephalon (sagittal view) 519 312 819 212:

1 — callosum 498 712 328 071

2 — pineal body (epiphysis) 519 317 819 217

3 — cerebellum 828 219 328 299

4 — medulla oblongata (myelencephalon) 519 211 068 001

5 — rhombencephalon 519 312 819 212

6 — pons 519 317 819 313

7 — pituitary (hypophysis) 317 218 219 819

8 — infundibulum 519 211 919 000

9 — optic chiasm 010 216 319 517

10 — hypothalamus 918 671 818 971

11 — interthalamic adhesion 248 719 361 989

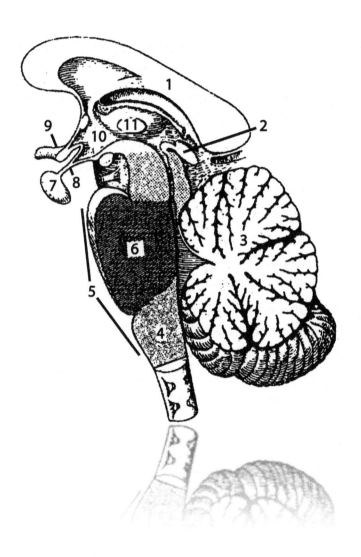

MENINGES (BRAIN MEMBRANES) 519 317 819 217

Fig. 22. Meninges (Brain membranes) 519 317 819 217:

1 — arachnoid granulation 514 312 814 712

2 — emissary vein 519 012 919 722

3 — diploic vein (vein of the spongy substance of bone) 518 712 318 222

4 — dura mater 333 489 312 289

5 — arachnoid trabeculae 519 317 919 227

6 — subarachnoid space 318 271 228 971

7 — choroid (cranial pia mater) 514 322 814 212

8 — arachnoid 319 217 064 827

9 — cerebral falx 001 918 021 378

10 — superior sagittal sinus 914 715 514 292

11 — cerebral cortex 918 617 619 017

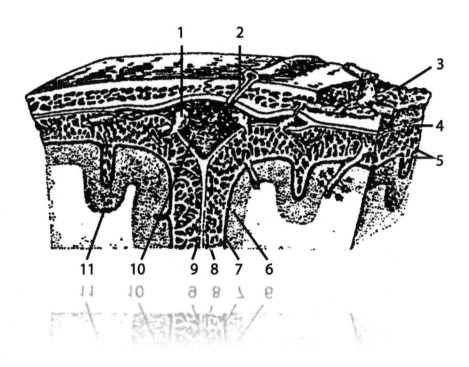

PERIPHERAL NERVOUS SYSTEM 519 555 819 915

CRANIAL NERVES 814 212 314 812

Fig. 23. Olfactory nerve 219 312 819 212:

1 — olfactory bulbs 917 318 219 518

2 — olfactory nerves 219 312 819 212

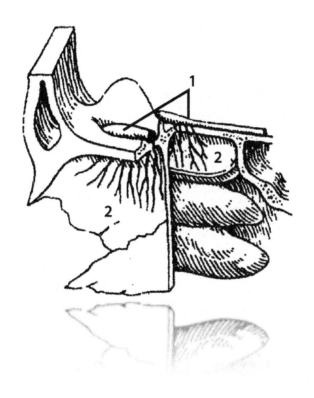

Fig. 24. Optic nerve 519 318 819 212:

1 — eyeball 519 321 819 288

2 — optic nerve 519 318 819 212

3 — orbital part 219 316 019 517

4 — intracanal part 514 317 814 218

5 — intracranial part 219 321 919 821

6 — optic chiasm 559 312 889 212

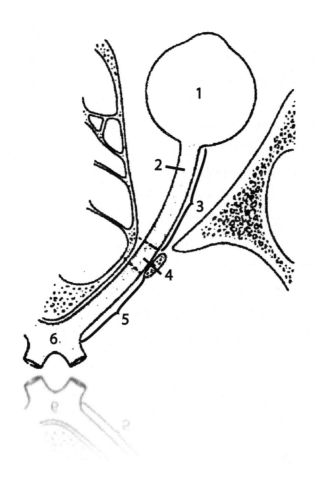

Fig. 25. Oculomotor and trochlear nerves 819 321 919 821:

1 — decussation of trochlear nerves 519 819 210 248

2 — trochlear nerve 551 478 984 512

3 — oculomotor 519 817 459 227

4 — sympathetic root 548 571 918 221

5 — part of optic nerve 514 812 214 022

6 — short ciliary nerves 478 521 928 321

7 — ciliary ganglion 519 788 589 228

8 — inferior branch of the oculomotor nerve 219 888 999 617

9 — nasal ciliary root 519 512 879 002

10 — trigeminal nerve 489 555 000 048

11 — superior branch of oculomotor nerve 501 048 998 118

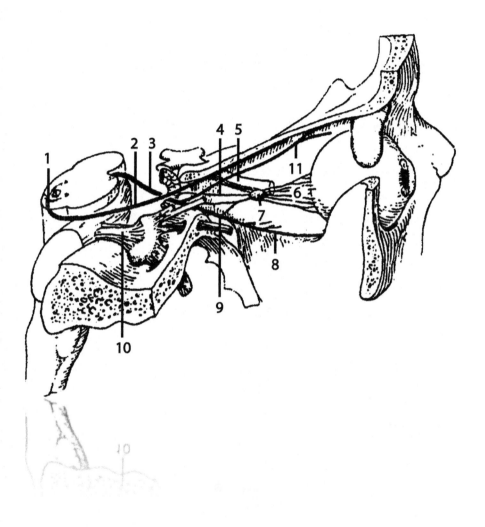

Fig. 26. Ophthalmic nerve

(first branch of trigeminal nerve) 914 815 914 715:

1 — motor rool 929 317 918 817

2 — tentorial membranous branch of nerve 929 317 918 513

3 — optic nerve 317 918 478 217

4 — frontal nerve 519 712 919 812

5 — supraorbital nerve 948 517 218 557

6 — communicating branch with zygomatic nerve 514 827 918 527

7 — optic nerve 519 312 819 212

8 — lacrimal nerve 478 217 378 217

9 — nasociliary nerve 519 318 219 298

10 — trigeminal ganglion 519 318 719 216

11 — trigeminal nerve 418 751 219 221

12 — sensory root 514 321 814 721

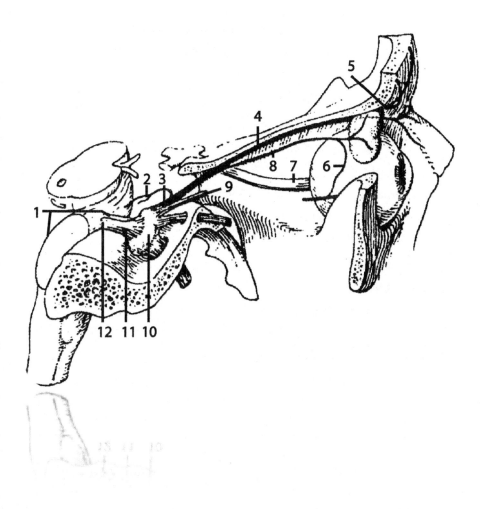

Fig. 27. Maxillary nerve (second branch of trigeminal nerve) 519 712 819 222:

1 — maxillary nerve 519 712 919 222

2 — zygomatic nerve 498 517 018 917

3 — infraorbital nerve 514 312 814 212

4 — lower branches of eyelids (palpebral branches) 519 231 919 811

5 — external nasal branches 519 817 919 227

6 — internal nasal branches 498 515 918 225

7 — upper labial branches 514 273 518 223

8 — upper dental branches 519 816 319 777

9 — upper gingival branches 418 217 918 227

10 — superior dental plexus 519 621 978 911

11 — middl upper alveolar branch 514 371 948 211

12 — posterior superior alveolar branches 514 327 549 247

13 — frontal superior alveolar branches 548 217 217 319

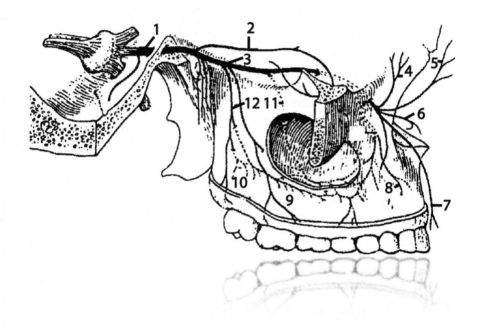

Fig. 28. Mandibular nerve (third branch of trigeminal nerve) 514 321 814 221:

1 — mandibular nerve 514 321 814 221

2 — lateral pterygoid nerve 214 712 814 212

3 — medial pterygoid nerve 519 712 819 212

4 — buccal nerve 514 312 814 212

5 — masseteric nerve 518 217 918 227

6 — auriculotemporal nerve 319 721 919 221

7 — anterior auricular nerves 248 655 448 755

8 — superficial temporal branches 429 321 899 411

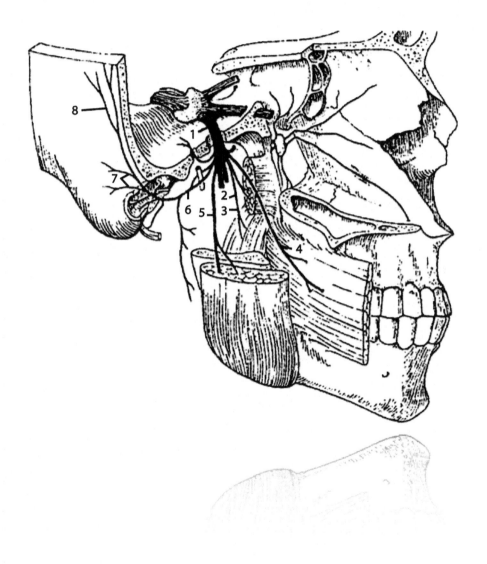

Fig. 29. Lingual nerve 214 318 714 818:

1 — lingual nerve 214 318 714 818

2 — mylohyoid nerve 519 312 419 712

3 — lingual branches 819 418 519 718

4 — sublingual nerve 531 418 818 819

5 — submandibular parasympathetic ganglion 314 815 214 915

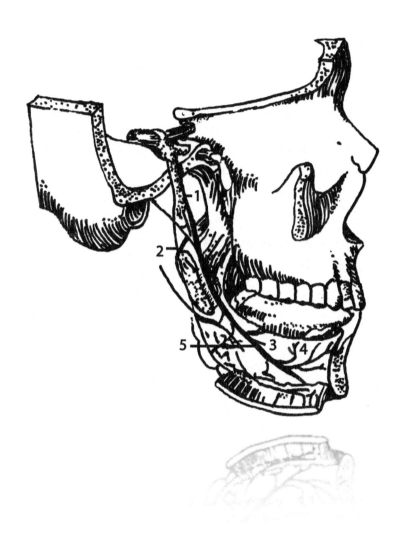

Fig. 30. Inferior alveolar nerve 891 318 519 458:

1 — lower alveolar nerve 519 314 818 888

2 — mylohyoid nerve 319 068 468 001

3 — mental nerve 319 814 819 914

4 — labial and gingival branches 514 813 914 608

5 — mental branches 319 812 819 312

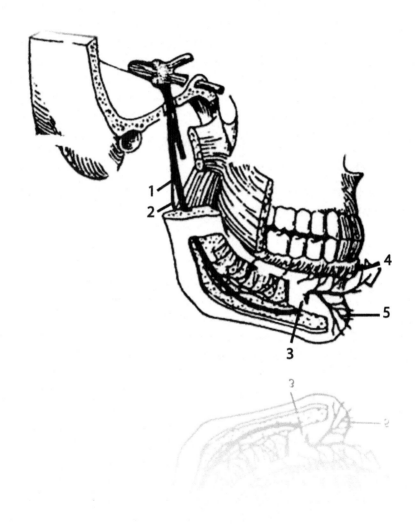

Fig. 31. ***Abducent nerve 513 428 913 918:***

1 — abducent nerve 513 428 913 918

2 — optic nerve 514 817 914 317

3 — bulbar muscles 548 712 818 912

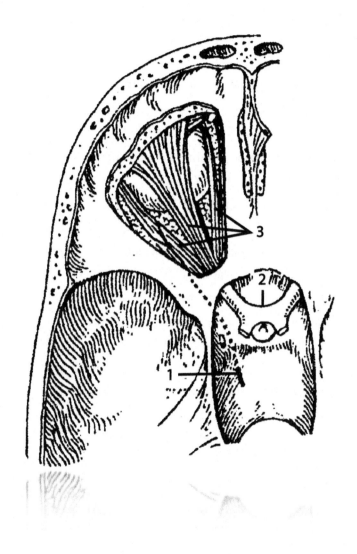

Fig. 32. Facial nerve 814 312 814 912:

1 — fundus of IV ventricle (rhomboid fossa) 519 318 010 624

2 — core of the facial nerve 668 317 918 517

3 — stylomastoid aperture (foramen) 514 318 214 818

4 — branch to the posterior ear (auricularis) muscle 919 312 819 512

5 — branch to the posterior belly of the digastric muscle 519 318 918 312

6 — branch to the stylohyoid muscle 514 812 819 412

7 — branches of the facial nerve to the mimetic muscles and subcutaneous muscle of the neck 514 317 418 219

8 — branch to the muscle lowering the angle of mouth (depressor muscle of angle of mouth) 514 317 214 317

9 — branch to the mental muscle 919 512 418 712

10 — branch to the muscle lowering the inferior lip 519 312 518 712

11 — branch to the buccal muscle (buccinator) 418 317 814 217

12 — branch to the orbicular muscle of mouth 219 379 891 472

13 — branch to the muscle lifting superior lip (levator muscle) 519 314 718 213

14 — branch to the zygomatic muscle 521 378 421 278

15 — branches to the orbicular muscle of eye 498 781 398 217

16 — branches to the frontal belly of epicranial muscle 548 371 898 217

17 — tympanichord (cord of tympanum) 519 712 891 421

18 — lingual nerve 214 318 714 818

19 — pterygopalatine ganglion 548 317 814 312

20 — trigeminus ganglion 517 819 319 218

21 — internal carotid artery 549 712 810 248

22 — intermediate nerve 548 317 218 227

23 — facial nerve 542 819 319 718

24 — vestibulocochlear nerve 528 317 228 487

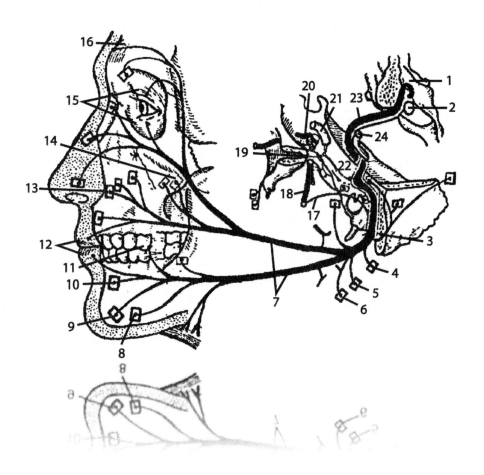

Fig. 33. Vestibulocochlear nerve 219 314 218 712:

1 — semicircular ducts 841 918 219 312

2 — lateral ampullar nerve 519 471 898 371

3 — anterior ampullar nerve 548 317 918 221

4 — utricular nerve 519 328 499 228

5 — utricular-ampullar nerve 514 312 814 882

6 — vestibular ganglion 719 317 919 817

7 — vestibular nerve 519 481 919 371

8 — vestibulocochlear nerve 518 317 918 221

9 — saccular nerve 518 472 918 222

10 — cochlear ganglion (spiral ganglion of cochlea) 914 712 814 212

11 — posterior ampullary nerve 219 473 218 223

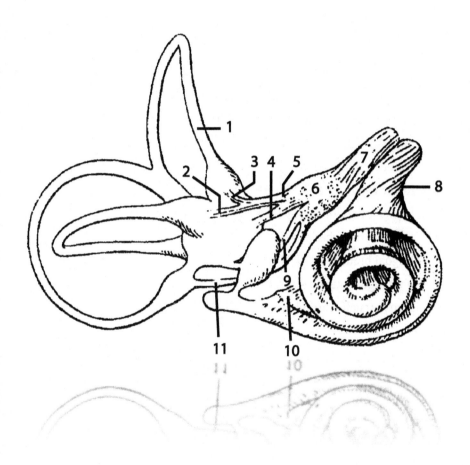

Fig. 34. Glossopharyngeal nerve 519 514 319 814:

1 — glossopharyngeal nerve 519 514 319 814

2 — upper ganglion 319 814 919 814

3 — connecting branch 519 317 068 007

4 — lower ganglion 319 216 519 428

5 — branch of stylopharyngeal muscle 542 718 212 328

6 — tonsillar branches 549 317 229 327

7 — lingual branches 819 418 519 718

8 — pharyngeal branch 498 217 228 417

9 — sinus branch (carotid branch) 319 421 219 221

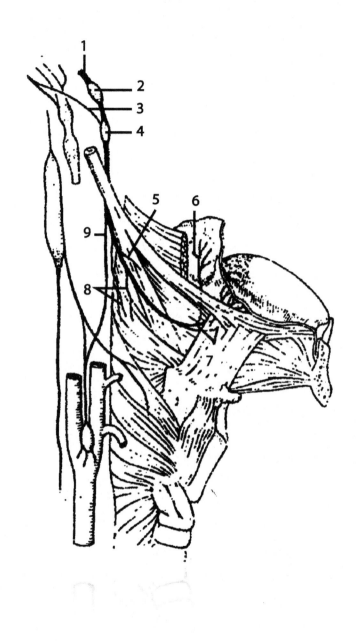

Fig. 35. Vagus nerve 489 981 728 221:

1 — vagus nerve 489 981 728 221

2 — upper ganglion 214 312 218 712

3 — lower ganglion 319 216 519 428

4 — meningeal branch 514 317 814 227

5 — aural nerve (auricular branch) 519 318 919 287

6 — connecting branch 519 321 919 811

7 — pharyngeal branches 498 217 998 897

8 — pharyngeal plexus 519 315 919 885

9 — upper cervical cardiac branches 498 712 319 882

10 — upper laryngeal nerve 498 882 319 982

11 — external branch 519 831 918 281

12 — internal branch 498 215 298 195

13 — connecting branch with recurrent laryngeal nerve 514 312 814 712

14 — lower cervical cardiac branches 498 761 998 251

15 — recurrent laryngeal nerve 518 472 888 912

16 — tracheal branches 919 810 499 310

17 — esophageal branches 519 512 319 812

18 — lower laryngeal nerve 514 312 814 222

19 — connecting branch with internal laryngeal branch 519 321 718 221

20 — thoracic cardiac branches 989 312 918 212

21 — bronchial branches 619 321 819 221

22 — pulmonary plexus 428 317 888 917

23 — esophageal plexus 219 317 819 227

24 — anterior vagal trunk 214 217 914 817

25 — posterior vagal trunk 219 317 219 228

26 — anterior gastric branches 289 317 299 277

27 — posterior gastric branches 298 312 678 212

28 — hepatic branches 214 213 219 312

29 — coeliac branches 298 012 718 202

30 — renal branches 219 317 209 717

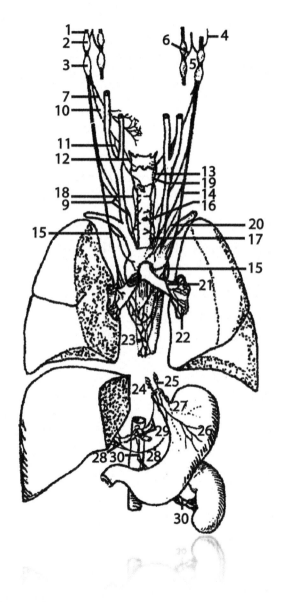

Fig. 36. Accessory nerve 519 312 819 222:

1 — spinal roots 428 713 228 213

2 — cranial roots (vagal part) 548 217 319 227

3 — trunk of accessory nerve 519 312 819 222

4 — internal branch 219 317 228 067

5 — external branch 519 387 219 277

6 — muscular branches 214 312 814 282

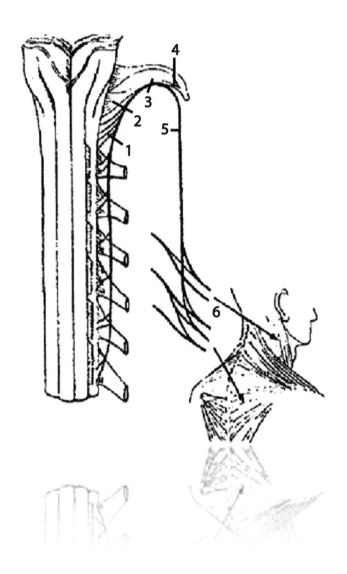

Fig. 37. Sublingual nerve and
cervical (sublingual) ansa 214 332 817 728:

1 — sublingual nerve 214 392 817 721

2 — thyrohyoid branch 519 513 419 213

3 — aterior root 519 317 819 228

4 — posterior root 409 272 819 322

5 — cervical (sublingual) ansa 841 332 817 798

6 — lingual branches 548 317 228 987

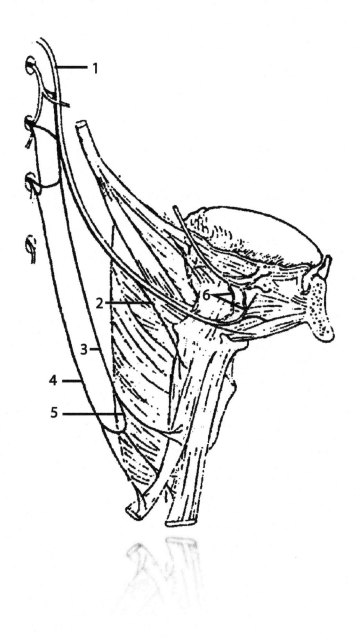

SPINAL NERVES 248 312 888 202

Fig. 38. Spinal nerve 248 312 888 202:

1 — trunk of spinal nerve 848 312 888 202

2 — anterior (motor) root 248 317 881 204

3 — posterior (sensitive) root 512 312 489 202

4 — root filaments 514 327 988 189

5 — spinal (sensitive) ganglion 918 312 889 202

6 — medial part of posterior branch 819 317 228 227

7 — lateral part of posterior branch 519 312 819 272

8 — posterior branch 548 715 888 215

9 — anterior branch 514 317 814 227

10 — white branch 518 714 318 214

11 — grey branch 229 829 318 912

12 — meningeal branch 498 517 328 777

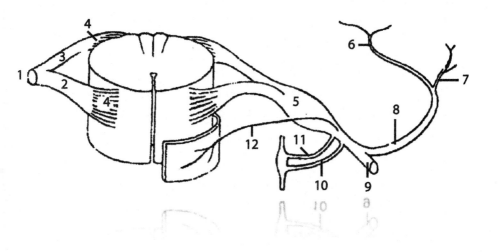

Fig. 39. Brachial plexus 312 314 512 214:

1 — diaphragmatic nerve (phrenic nerve) 519 378 219 888

2 — dorsal nerve of scapula 888 888 919 017

3 — upper trunk of bronchial plexus 428 217 228 277

4 — middle trunk of bronchial plexus 514 312 814 222

5 — subclavian trunk 498 217 289 277

6 — lower trunk of bronchial plexus 748 213 888 213

7 — accessory diaphragmatic nerves 067 214 327 224

8 — long thoracic nerve 519 312 819 222

9 — medial thoracic nerve 418 722 888 222

10 — lateral thoracic nerve 214 317 914 777

11 — medial fascicle 819 312 819 314

12 — posterior fascicle 889 212 478 312

13 — lateral fascicle 514 312 889 212

14 — suprascapular nerve 418 319 218 912

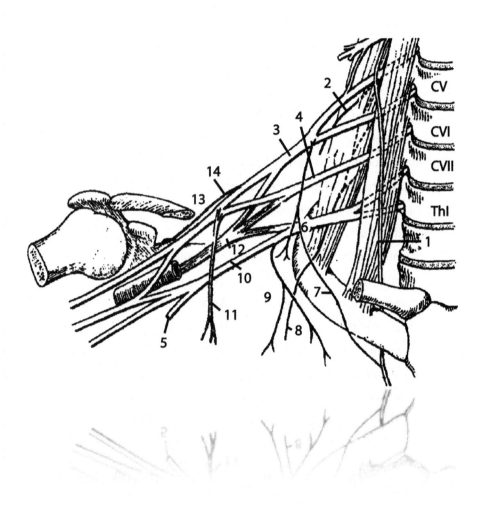

CV
CVI
CVII
ThI

Fig. 40. Nerves of shoulder, forearm and hand 412 818 219 314:

A — nerves of shoulder 514 312 814 212:

1 — medial cutaneous nerve of shoulder and medial cutaneous nerve of forearm 428 312 518 212

2 — median nerve 498 717 818 217

3 — shoulder artery 514 312 814 212

4 — ulnar nerve 319 817 919 016

5 — biceps muscle of arm (distal end) 519 312 819 222

6 — radial nerve 514 317 814 212

7 — shoulder muscle (brachialis) 319 717 819 317

8 — musculocutaneous nerve 512 314 212 814

9 — biceps muscle of arm (proximal end) 514 217 914 317

B — nerves of forearm and hand 218 001 209 317:

1 — median nerve 518 519 318 219

2 — round pronator (transected) muscle 214 888 219 317

3 — ulnar nerve 218 312 418 222

4 — deep flexor muscle of fingers (flexor digitorum profundus) 213 814 818 217

5 — anterior interosseous nerve 548 312 819 272

6 — dorsal branch of ulnar nerve 428 577 928 227

7 — deep branch of ulnar nerve 458 317 218 757

8 — superficial branch of ulnar nerve 419 312 819 422

9 — quadrate pronator muscle (transected) 428 317 228 917

10 — superficial branch of radial nerve 548 217 328 227

11 — brachioradial muscle (transected) 429 318 229 718

12 — radial nerve 514 321 558 221

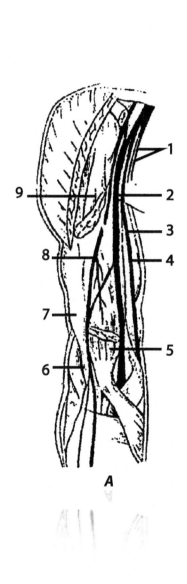

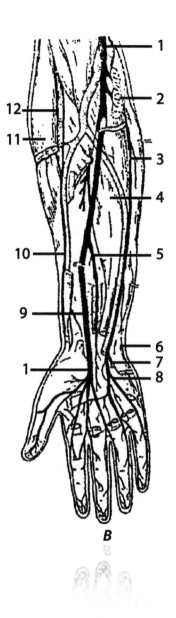

A   B

Fig. 41. Lumbosacral plexus 214 712 814 328:

1 — posterior branches of lumbar nerves 418 712 818 322

2 — anterior branches of lumbar nerves 514 372 814 222

3 — iliohypogastric nerve 514 371 814 211

4 — genitofemoral nerve 518 317 989 316

5 — ilioinguinal nerve 514 317 814 217

6 — lateral cutaneous nerve of thigh 519 618 919 818

7 — femoral branch 514 317 814 818

8 — genital branch 528 712 328 912

9 — anterior scrotal nerves 428 319 718 219

10 — anterior branch of obturator nerve 514 718 219 317

11 — obturator nerve 589 317 919 217

12 — lumbosacral plexus 214 712 814 328

13 — anterior branches of sacral plexus 548 312 219 228

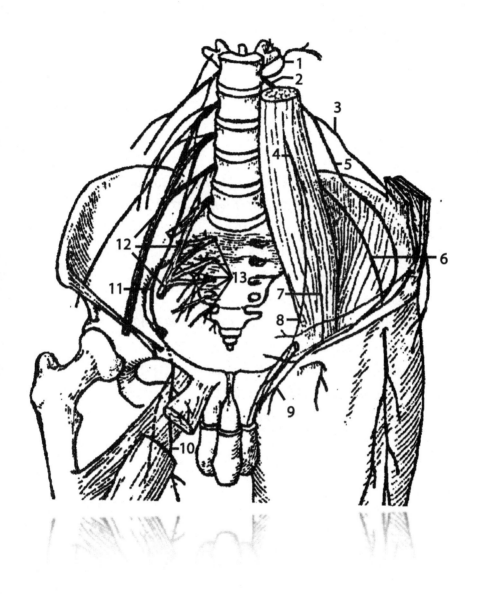

Fig. 42. Nerves of gluteal region and
posterior surface of thigh 214 718 219 312:

1 — upper gluteal nerve 419 715 819 215

2 — sciatic nerve 898 919 719 828

3, 4 — muscle branches of sciatic nerve 214 312 814 712

5 — tibial nerve 518 714 818 914

6 — common peroneal (fibular) nerve 498 217 998 717

7 — lateral cutaneous nerve of calf 492 517 212 817

8 — posterior cutaneous nerve of thigh 514 317 218 277

9 — lower gluteal nerve 819 215 518 225

10 — medial dorsal cutaneous nerve 514 312 814 872

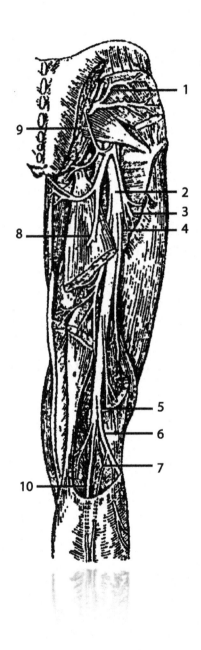

Fig. 43. Nerves of shin (posterior surface) 548 217 218 887:

1 — sciatic nerve 513 418 213 918

2 — common peroneal (fibular) nerve 514 312 814 522

3 — tibial nerve 514 812 919 222

4, 7, 8 — muscle branches of tibial nerve 548 714 818 214

5 — lateral cutaneous nerve of calf 498 217 318 717

6 — muscle branches of peroneal nerve 548 219 319 878

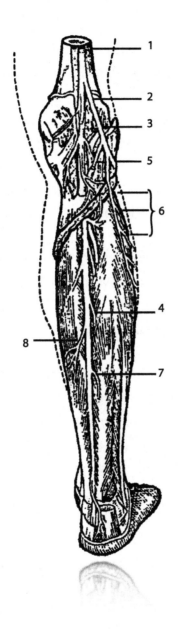

VEGETATIVE (AUTONOMOUS) NERVOUS SYSTEM 514 312 819 981

SYMPATHETIC PART OF VEGETATIVE (AUTONOMOUS) NERVOUS SYSTEM 891 418 318 888

PARASYMPATHETIC PART OF VEGETATIVE (AUTONOMOUS) NERVOUS SYSTEM 418 217 318 918

CYTOARCHITECTONIC CORTICAL AREAS OF LARGE CEREBRAL HEMISPHERES 219 047 819 215

Fig. 44. Reflex arch 219 317 819 892:

1 — nerve endings of sensitive neuron in skin 428 317 918 217

2 — peripheral process of sensitive neuron 519 317 919 817

3 — neurit of motor cell 428 312 918 212

4 — nerve ending in muscle 519 317 918 287

5 — motor cell of anterior horn 491 218 519 328

6 — intercalated neuron 428 317 918 219

7 — central process of sensitive neuron 512 216 219 327

8 — spinal ganglion 428 312 219 217

SIGNAL SYSTEMS 891 312 918 412

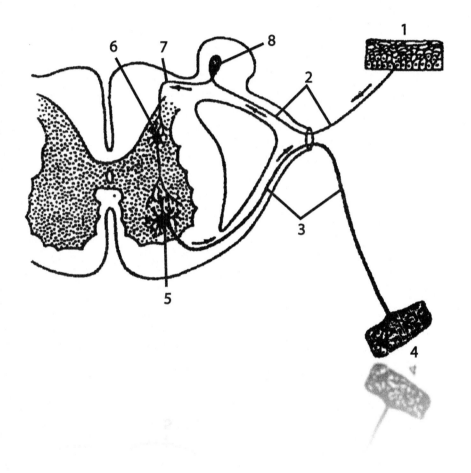

SENSE ORGANS 214 712 514 312

ORGAN OF VISION 219 317 989 312

Fig. 45. Eye 514 317 814 917:

1 — sclera 928 317 818 917

2 — choroid 218 712 819 312

3 — retina 319 218 918 217

4 — Central pit 514 312 814 212

5 — blind spot 489 000 909 216

6 — optic nerve 487 321 481 519

7 — conjunctiva 528 317 312 819

8 — ciliary ligament 898 312 519 482

9 — cornea 489 317 219 217

10 — pupil 489 319 218 213

11, 18 — optical axis 519 317 419 817

12 — anterior chamber 428 312 818 212

13 — lens 519 321 819 221

14 — iris 428 218 318 219

15 — posterior chamber 489 312 918 216

16 — ciliary muscle 219 312 719 312

17 — hyaline 519 322 819 212

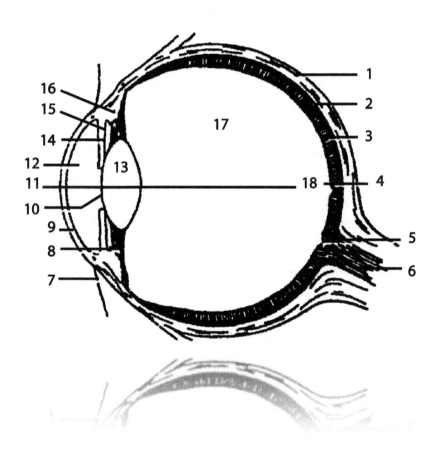

Fig. 46. Muscles of eyeball 512 901 318 201:

A — view from the lateral side:

1 — superior rectus 219 317 218 227

2 — muscle lifting upper eyelid 512 419 312 228

3 — inferior oblique muscle 219 317 819 227

4 — inferior rectus muscle 219 317 219 827

5 — lateral rectus muscle 328 421 898 712

B — view form above:

1 — trochlea 229 457 298 788

2 — tendon sheath of superior oblique muscle 248 272 458 299

3 — superior oblique muscle 219 312 919 802

4 — medial rectus muscle 898 782 988 312

5 — inferior rectus muscle 219 317 219 827

6 — superior rectus muscle 219 317 218 227

7 — lateral rectus muscle 328 421 898 712

8 — muscle lifting the upper eyelid 512 419 312 228

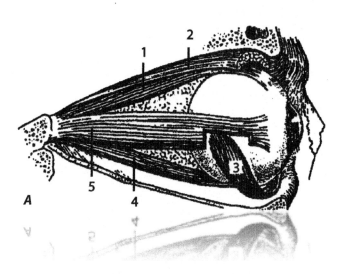

A

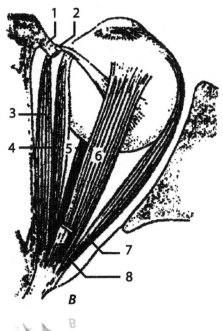

B

Fig. 47. visual analyzer 219 318 719 817:

1 — retina 319 218 918 217

2 — uncrossed fibers of optic nerve 214 317 819 007

3 — crossed fibers of optic nerve 719 300 800 111

4 — optic tract 419 916 819 317

5 — cortical analyzer 519 312 819 227

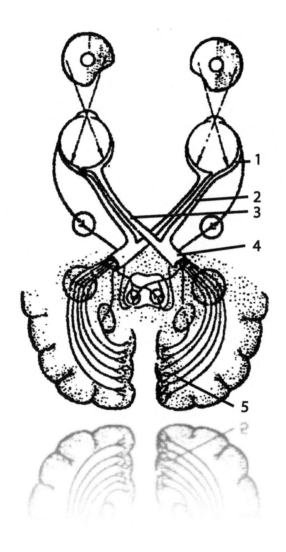

ORGAN OF AUDITION AND EQUILIBRIUM 248 712 318 222

Fig. 48. vestibulocochlear organ
(organ of audition and equilibrium) 248 712 318 222:

1 — superior semicircular duct 498 312 818 221

2 — vestibule 948 218 298 820

3 — cochlea 321 018 204 516

4 — auditory nerve 458 912 312 819

5 — carotid artery 428 713 828 213

6 — auditory tube 429 318 919 228

7 — tympanic cavity 519 317 919 827

8 — tympanic membrane 429 317 229 817

9 — external auditory meatus 519 421 919 811

10 — external auditory pore 521 917 319 817

11 — auricle 421 918 518 717

12 — malleus 521 328 421 891

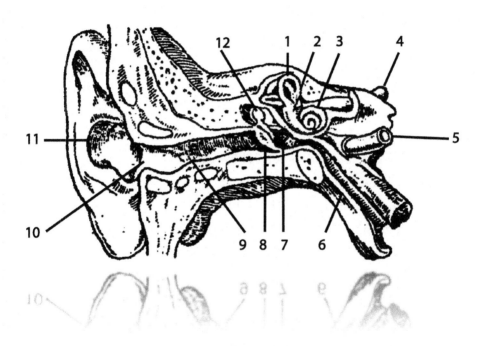

Fig. 49. Auditory ossicles 428 317 218 227:

1 — incudomalleal joint 214 312 914 212

2 — short crus of incus 512 612 218 377

3 — body of incus 889 891 892 712

4 — incus 521 488 711 918

5 — long crus of incus 548 712 528 312

6 — lenticular process 528 219 312 219

7 — posterior crus of stapes 428 517 928 717

8 — stapes 498 714 889 216

9 — base of stapes 378 819 498 881

10 — anterior crus of stapes 488 711 294 301

11 — head of stapes 481 499 816 701

12 — incudostapedial joint 797 014 398 481

13 — manubrium of malleus 878 421 891 216

14 — anterior process of malleus 219 054 398 716

15 — lateral process of malleus 481 898 714 849

16 — malleus 521 328 421 891

17 — neck of malleus 891 219 311 919

18 — head of malleus 214 312 814 918

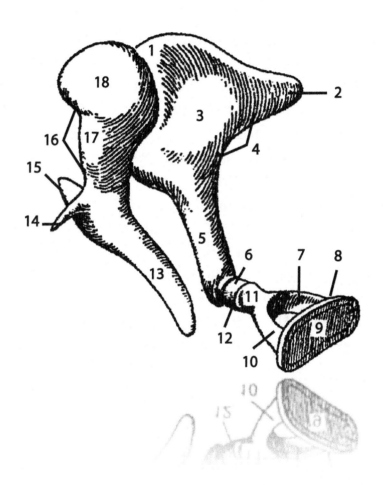

Fig. 50. Cochlear canal (crosscut view):

1 — vestibular canal 219 317 918 516

2 — vestibular wall of the cochlear duct 214 712 814 312

3 — tectorial membrane 498 516 679 210

4 — cochlear duct 312 814 219 322

5 — auditory cells with cilia 512 418 622 898

6 — supporting cells 548 312 988 822

7 — spiral ridge (spiral ligament) 528 318 618 227

8 — bone tissue of cochlear 428 219 319 891

9 — supporting cell 219 214 319 814

10 — Corti's cells-pillars 214 316 719 816

11 — tympanic canal of cochlea 918 421 519 317

12 — basilar plate 514 321 898 218

13 — nerve cells of the spiral ganglion 428 317 428 527

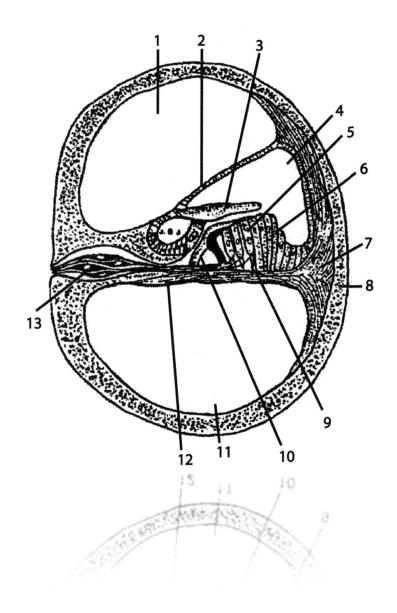

GUSTATORY ORGAN 419 317 819 227

Fig. 51. lingual papilla.
Gustatory areas of tongue 419 381 489 294:

A — lingual papilla 419 381 489 294

a — general look 914 819 319 821

b — fungiform papilla 314 218 914 888

c — filiform papilla 514 317 814 217

d — foliate papilla 428 312 818 212

e — vallate papilla 219 214 319 814

    (1 — fungiform papilla 314 218 914 888

    2 — filiform papilla 514 317 814 217

    3 — foliate papilla 428 312 818 212

    4 — vallate papilla 219 214 319 814)

B — Gustatory areas of tongue 419 317 819 217

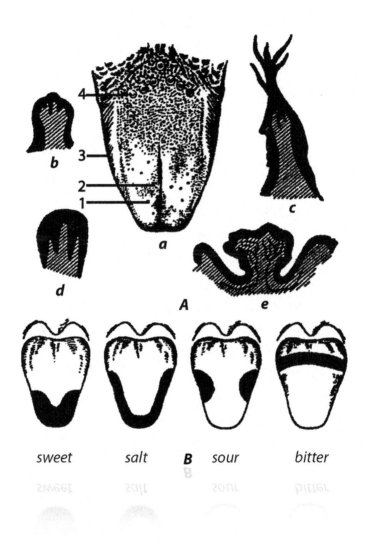

4 —
3 —
2 —
1 —

b

a

c

d

A

e

sweet   *salt*   **B** *sour*   *bitter*

OLFACTORY ORGAN 914 782 214 389
SKIN 519 606 901 319

Fig. 52. Human skin: (A - crosscut view;
B – visible structures) 519 606 901 319:

1 — granular layer 514 317 814 297

2 — corneal layer 548 671 918 311

3 — spinous layer 914 917 414 897

4 — hair follicle 314 912 814 889

5 — sebaceous glands 498 791 229 321

6 — secretory cells 519 818 229 398

7 — sweat gland 519 488 598 719

8 — gland duct 891 098 789 016

9 — hair papilla 918 781 298 391

10 — subcutaneous fat cells 898 712 918 312

11 — subcutaneous tissue 519 861 719 211

12 — part of the hair rod 598 061 214 711

13 — blood vessel 217 918 294 888

14 — dermis 498 718 519 317

15 — elastic and collagen fibers 519 618 718 215

16 — epidermis 598 718 889 888

Numerical concentrations on skin stimulate recovery of the matter in conjunction with the entire organism. Separation of the internal space of organism and the external space in relation to the body allows numerical concentrations on the skin of the body to operate the organism events and outside of it wider than numerical concentrations for other matter. That is why it is possible to implement skin concentrations as an accelerating element in event operation. Micro and macro objects which are harmful to the body, including infections and so on, can be removed faster from the body or obstructed from lesions of organism using numerical concentrations on skin.

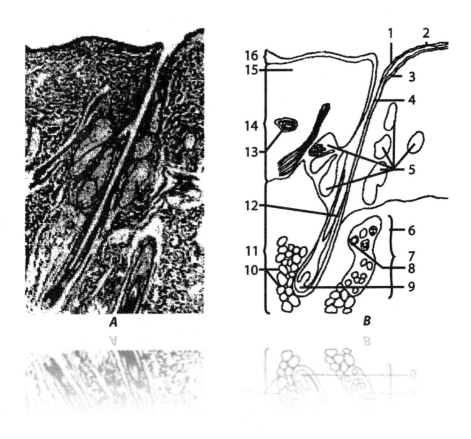

BONES 214 318 214 818

BONES JUNCTIONS 814 312 214 712

Fig. 53. Types of bones junctions:

A — joint 314 812 514 212

B — fibrous junction 719 312 819 212

C — synchondrosis (cartilaginous joint) 314 217 914 818

D — symphysis 319 812 919 212

1 — periosteum 514 312 814 712

2 — bone 418 517 918 217

3 — fibrous connective tissue 519 318 219 417

4 — cartilage 314 217 914 819

5 — synovial membrane 214 317 914 817

6 — fibrous membrane 319 217 916 074

7 — articular cartilage 314 217 914 914

8 — articular cavity 312 817 918 217

9 — fissure in interpubic disk 514 318 217 218

10 — interpubic disk 219 312 219 212

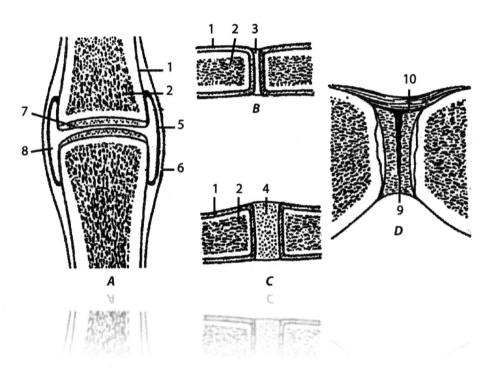

TORSO SKELETON 219 314 819 217

Fig. 54. Human skeleton 219 317 918 428:

1 — skul 519 515 919 894

2 — spinal column 328 488 984 012

3 — collarbone 409 382 984 712

4 — rib 519 312 918 722

5 — sternum 518 417 289 897

6 — humerus 524 377 914 877

7 — radius 529 321 919 742

8 — ulnar bone 529 341 419 811

9 — carpal bones 318 712 918 212

10 — metacarpals 214 371 814 911

11 — phalanges 548 317 918 217

12 — ilium 218 317 228 917

13 — sacrum 514 716 814 226

14 — pubic bone 512 478 212 238

15 — ischial bone 498 216 748 227

16 — femoral bone 918 275 784 325

17 — patella 421 891 529 328

18 — tibia 918 321 989 711

19 — fibula 498 217 888 917

20 — tarsal bones 498 215 298 315

21 — metatarsals 494 216 894 317

22 — phalanges of the foot 548 321 984 671

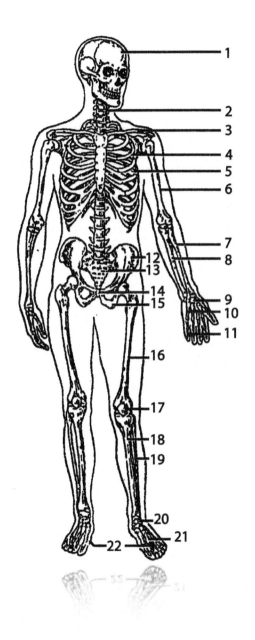

Fig. 55. Cervical vertebra 219 213 319 721:

1 — superior articular process 519 317 819 217

2 — arc vertebra 519 312 919 212

3 — vertebral foramen 514 312 214 712

4 — spinal process 548 312 848 212

5 — plate vertebral arch 517 218 317 918

6 — inferior articular process 517 919 217 398

7 — posterior tubercle 514 317 814 917

8 — groove of spinal nerve 219 317 819 218

9 — foramen transverse process 514 318 218 214

10 — anterior bump 519 218 218 914

11 — vertebral body 317 689 318 918

12 — uncus of body 519 312 819 212

13 — transverse process 514 312 814 912

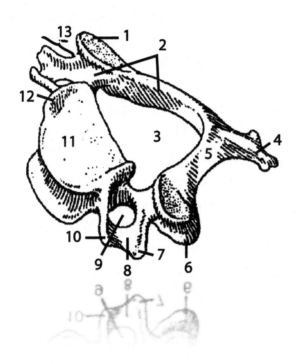

Fig. 56. Thoracic vertebrae 219 214 319 814:

1 — limb of arch vertebra 498 317 218 217

2 — superior vertebral notch 214 312 814 712

3, 7 — transverse process 519 317 819 217

4 — superior articular process 219 715 319 215

5, 9 — upper rib fossa 549 312 814 212

6 — the spinal canal 521 314 818 214

8 — spinal process 319 712 819 212

10 — costal fovea of transverse process 821 319 921 819

11 — inferior articular process 419 312 819 212

12 — inferior vertebral notch 512 314 812 214

13, 14 — inferior costal fossa 019 712 219 312

15 — vertebral body 519 317 819 217

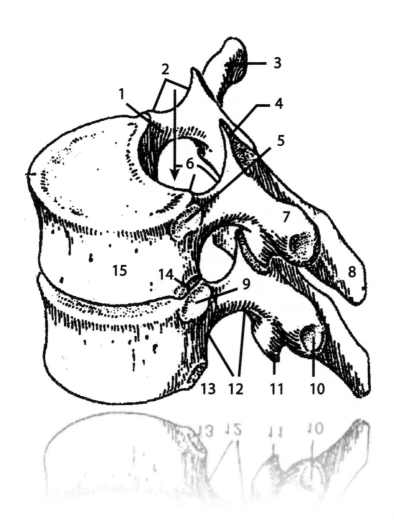

Fig. 57. Lumbar vertebra (top view) 519 317 819 218:

1 — spinal process 513 219 813 919

2 — superior articular process 419 712 819 212

3 — costal process 317 814 214 917

4 — arc vertebra 519 312 819 212

5 — vertebral foramen 828 317 918 217

6 — limb of arch vertebra 498 317 218 227

7 — vertebral body 519 317 819 227

8 — accessory process 518 431 219 917

9 — mammillary process 519 817 919 217

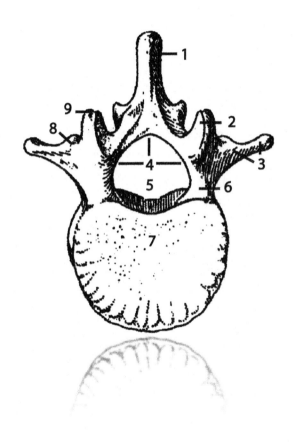

Fig. 58. Sacrum (front view) 548 312 218 312:

1 — base of sacrum 548 317 218 227

2 — superior articular process 519 328 919 228

3 — anterior surface of sacrum 549 218 319 228

4 — transversal lines 428 213 328 333

5 — tip of the sacrum 408 217 229 327

6 — anterior sacral foramina 489 213 217 289

7 — promontory 428 327 828 227

8 — lateral part 319 712 919 212

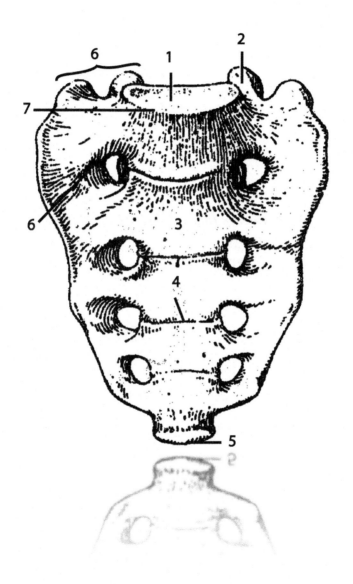

Fig. 59. Coccyx (back view) 519 513 819 213;

1 — coccyx 519 513 819 213

2 — coccygeal horn 514 717 814 317

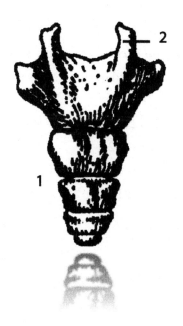

Fig. 60. The first and second rib (top view) 214 712 814 312:

1 — articular surface of the head of rib 512 318 912 218

2 — head of rib 214 718 218 214

3 — tubercle of rib 518 380 218 910

4 — body of rib 538 712 818 222

5 — articular surface of the tubercle of rib 419 710 819 210

6 — neck of rib 498 217 218 317

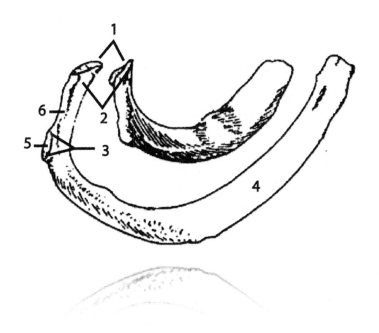

Fig. 61. Seventh rib (inner surface) 519 318 919 218:

1 — articular surface of the head of rib 514 312 814 212

2 — articular surface of the tubercle of rib 519 317 819 217

3 — tubercle of rib 518 714 318 214

4 — neck of rib 419 712 819 212

5 — angle of rib 219 718 218 312

6 — body of rib 217 419 218 219

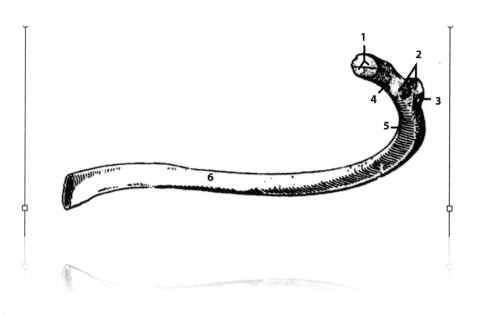

Fig. 62. Vertebral column 214 217 000 819:

1 — cervical vertebrae 312 218 212 918

2 — thoracic vertebrae 214 217 814 717

3 — lumbar vertebrae 498 217 218 227

4 — sacrum 213 819 222 218

5 — tailbone 218 312 248 228

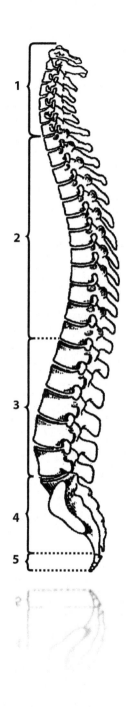

Fig. 63. Skeleton of chest (front view) 248 668 712 298:

1 — superior thoracic aperture 520 319 210 299

2 — jugular notch 548 717 818 997

3 — ribs (1—12) 431 898 211 328

4 — the first rib 317 814 217 214

5, 16 — the second rib 518 513 918 913

6 — manubrium of sternum 819 312 219 312

7 — body of sternum 514 318 219 217

8 — joint between the body of sternum and xiphoid
process 512 318 918 212

9 — xiphoid process 219 318 719 228

10 — oscillating ribs (11—12) 514 217 214 317

11 — false ribs (8—12) 548 212 228 312

12 — thoracic vertebra 542 317 212 227

13 — inferior thoracic aperture 009 217 819 317

14 — sternum 514 317 814 817

15 — true rib (1—7) 519 312 819 212

17 — clavicular notch 312 814 212 418

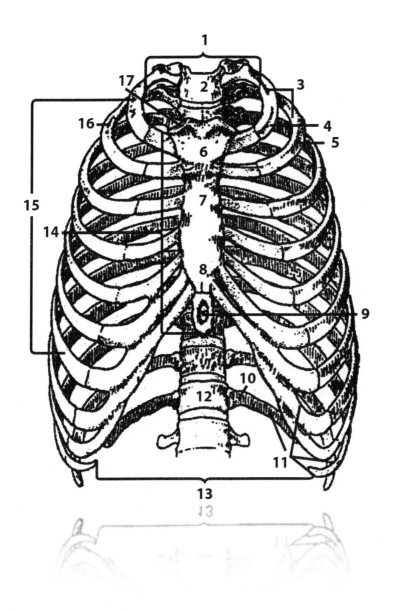

SKELETON HEAD 231 138 918 212

Fig. 64. Frontal bone 248 003 398 213:

1 — squama 214 317 818 217

2 — frontal tuber 219 317 818 227

3 — temporal line 248 312 298 222

4 — zygomatic process 248 714 318 214

5 — supraorbital margin 249 312 289 228

6 — supraorbital foramen 312 278 229 312

7 — nasal part 248 217 228 327

8 — glabella 814 712 214 312

9 — superciliary arch 428 517 228 917

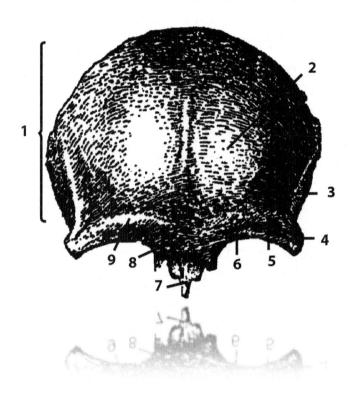

145

Fig. 65. Right parietal bone (inner surface) 312 718 212 218:

1 — sagittal edge 428 713 228 213

2 — rump aperture 312 219 218 271

3 — groove of superior sagittal sinus 214 317 228 271

4 — occipital angle 248 712 219 220

5 — occipital margin 319 714 219 514

6 — mastoid angle 314 217 214 227

7 — groove of sigmoid sinus 278 213 228 913

8 - 10 — furrow of middle meningeal artery 514 317 814 717

11 — wedge angle 594 018 294 318

12 — frontal margin 519 312 819 212

13 — inner surface 234 712 814 212

14 — frontal angle 514 001 814 321

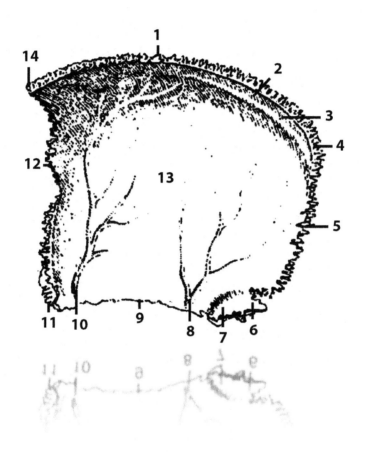

Fig. 66. Left parietal bone
(outer surface) 326 718 216 718:

1 — sagittal edge 519 312 819 213

2 — parietal hole 594 312 919 312

3 — occipital angle 528 317 818 227

4 — occipital margin 548 321 918 221

5 — superior temporal line 548 312 718 212

6 — mastoid angle 319 217 819 227

7 — squamous edge 298 714 888 914

8 — cuneate angle 548 712 219 312

9 — inferior temporal line 548 317 818 717

10 — frontal edge 514 718 214 318

11 — parietal protuberance 219 317 918 227

12 — the outer surface 519 318 719 288

13 — frontal angle 319 217 219 717

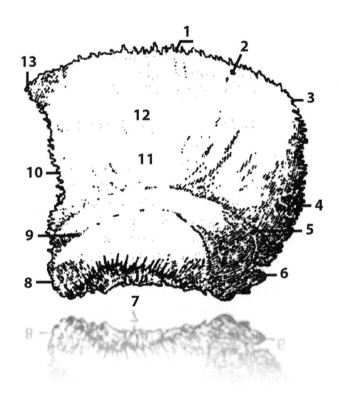

Fig. 67. Occipital bone (inner surface) 214 712 219 312:

1 — groove of superior sagittal sinus 518 317 918 919

2 — cerebral fossa 549 312 919 217

3 — occipital squama 598 317 919 217

4 — cruciform eminence 519 312 299 812

5 — internal occipital protuberance 312 818 712 918

6 — groove of transverse sinus 519 317 919 217

7 — internal occipital crest 514 715 914 315

8 — cerebellar fossa 219 213 919 223

9 — condylar canal 231 918 298 221

10 — jugular process 498 317 998 227

11 — large aperture 201 398 721 778

12 — jugular tubercle 548 715 328 225

13 — basilar part 549 713 919 223

14 — pharyngeal tubercle 548 712 228 312

15 — occipital condyle 549 317 819 223

16 — lateral part 549 717 229 237

17 — mastoid edge 542 713 222 203

18 — lambdoid edge 519 321 009 811

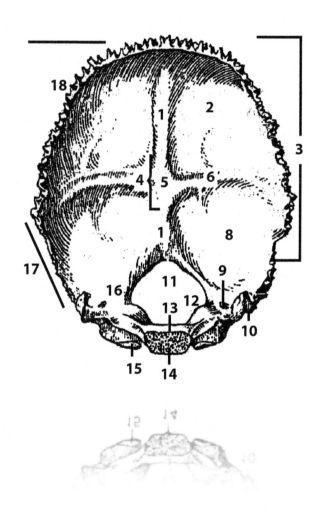

Fig. 68. Occipital bone (back and bottom view) 548 717 218 317:

1 — occipital squama 514 312 214 712

2 — jugular tubercle 548 715 328 225

3 — clivus 319 778 219 228

4 — large aperture 519 712 819 222

5 — condylar canal 319 713 819 223

6 — occipital condyle 519 715 819 225

7 — condylar fossa 539 812 918 222

8 — inferior nuchal line 514 701 814 321

9 — external occipital crest 514 312 814 722

10 — superior nuchal line 548 717 888 999

11 — the highest nuchal line 599 000 089 319

12 — occipital area 538 721 918 211

13 — external occipital protuberance 429 312 819 228

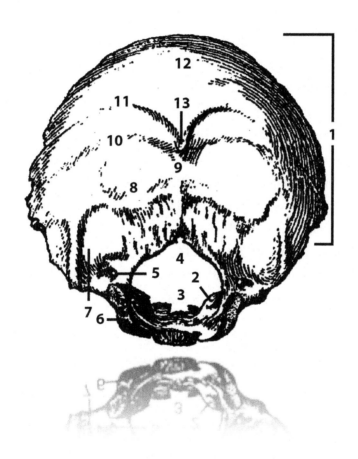

Fig. 69. cuneiform bone (top view) 219 317 919 227:

1 — lesser wing (left) 329 717 229 317

2 — body 429 811 319 321

3 — sulcus of chiasm 314 717 814 217

4 — pituitary fossa 519 317 919 218

5 — visual channel 538 712 918 222

6 — superior orbital fissure 409 505 898 305

7 — round aperture 319 712 819 222

8, 12 — large wings 217 318 917 228

9 — oval foramen 298 714 318 214

10 — spinous hole 219 542 319 712

11 — dorsum sellae 548 713 918 213

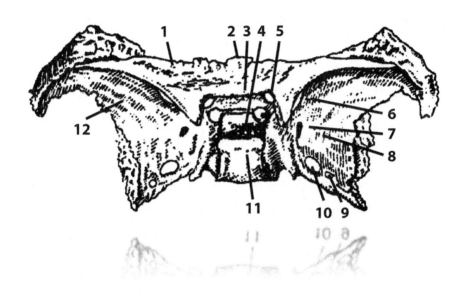

Fig. 70. Right temporal bone (inner surface) 549 317 914 317:

1 — upper edge of pyramid 219 317 919 227

2 — groove of superior petrosal sinus 549 312 819 229

3 — furrow of sigmoid sinus 098 174 219 314

4 — internal process 214 712 914 229

5 — jugular notch 531 918 911 218

6 — styloid process 598 312 818 212

7 — internal acoustic meatus 548 211 918 211

8 — internal auditory canal 531 988 411 888

9 — groove of inferior petrosal sinus 219 213 919 733

10 — posterior edge of pyramid 214 313 219 733

11 — posterior surface of pyramid 519 312 814 222

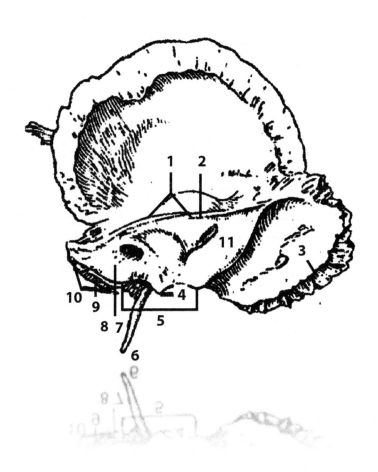

Fig. 71. Right temporal bone (outer surface) 519 312 419 812:

1 — tympanosquamous fissure 514 317 814 317

2 — petrotympanic fissure 548 321 948 221

3 — styloid process 398 213 998 223

4 — tympanomastoid fissure 598 712 898 223

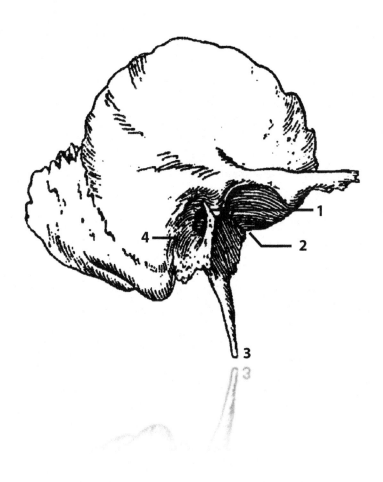

1

4

2

3

3

FACIAL BONES OF SKULL 219 715 819 815

Fig. 72. Maxilla (view from the lateral side) 519 371 919 811:

1 — orbital surface 398 216 718 226

2 — infraorbital furrow 319 717 819 227

3 — zygomatic process 419 312 214 222

4 — alveolar apertures 214 712 814 229

5 — subtemporal surface 538 722 918 222

6 — front surface 548 888 019 648

7 — fang fossa 539 717 819 317

8 — anterior nasal bone 529 513 919 813

9 — body of maxilla 548 712 818 212

10 — nasal incisure 519 312 819 212

11 — infraorbital canal 319 717 819 217

12 — infraorbital aperture 319 712 819 212

13 — zygomaticomaxillary suture 214 711 898 211

14 — frontal process 319 712 819 222

15 — lachrymal edge 548 884 918 888

16 — infraorbital edge 512 219 312 919

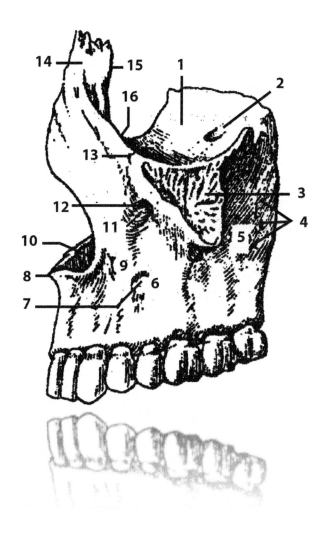

Fig. 73. Left upper jaw
(view from the medial side) 421 718 911 328:

1 — frontal process 428 317 228 917

2 — nasal surface 519 317 819 217

3 — anterior nasal spine 214 317 814 227

4 — palatine sulcus of palatine bone 428 321 814 221

5 — maxillary sinus 519 321 814 471

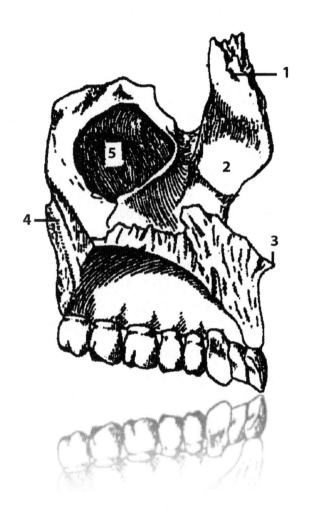

Fig. 74. Lower jaw 514 712 814 312:

1 — head of the lower jaw 548 321 848 721

2 — pterygoid fossa 519 317 919 007

3 — neck of the mandible 319 814 919 714

4, 5 — branches of the lower jaw 518 317 918 001

6 — angle of the mandible 548 219 289 008

7 — channel of the lower jaw 009 217 319 227

8 — temporal ridge 418 317 228 227

9 — aperture of the lower jaw 489 201 319 871

10 — coronoid process 528 317 918 228

11 — nasal incisure of the lower jaw 419 317 819 828

12 — condylar process 891 319 898 789

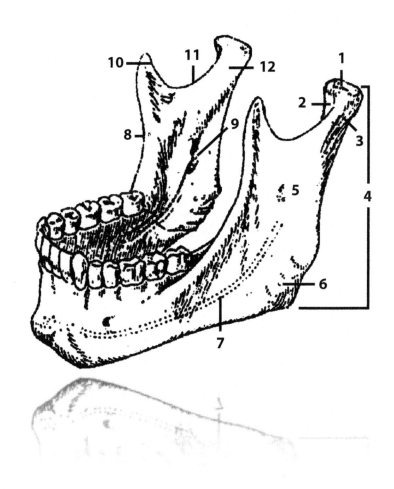

© Г.П. Грабовой 2002

165

Fig. 75. Human skull (front view) 829 317 229 817:

1 — coronal suture 419 289 917 814

2 — parietal bone 519 987 219 317

3 — orbital part of the frontal bone 998 261 378 471

4 — orbital surface of greater wing of sphenoid bone 548 261 378 213

5 — cheekbone 899 817 818 317

6 — inferior nasal concha 478 218 918 217

7 — upper jaw 521 718 221 918

8 — chin protrusion of the lower jaw 319 712 819 222

9 — nasal cavity 428 317 818 227

10 — vomer 429 317 819 228

11 — perpendicular plate of the ethmoid bone 219 317 819 227

12 — orbital surface of the upper jaw 428 712 818 212

13 — inferior orbital fissure 429 731 819 221

14 — lacrimal bone 209 605 319 205

15 — orbital plate of the ethmoid bone 398 667 818 917

16 — superior orbital fissure 409 505 898 305

17 — squamous part of temporal bone 428 319 288 299

18 — zygomatic process of frontal bone 319 712 819 212

19 — visual channel 498 712 818 222

20 — nasal bone 518 314 818 214

21 — frontal tuber 518 712 918 212

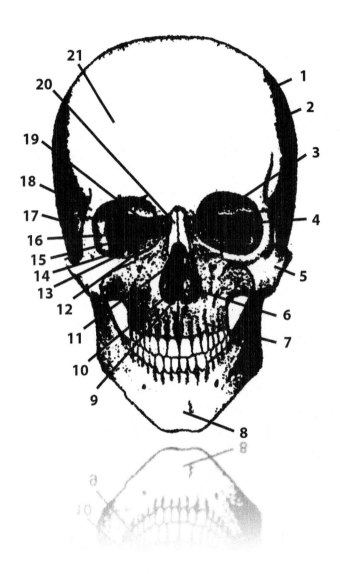

Fig. 76. Human skull (lateral view) 829 317 229 817:

1 — parietal bone 829 312 919 212

2 — coronal suture 428 317 928 777

3 — frontal tuber 719 317 819 217

4 — temporal surface of greater wing of cuneiform bone 514 317 049 612

5 — orbital plate of the ethmoid bone 518 714 318 914

6 — lacrimal bone 967 912 319 812

7 — nasal bone 519 314 819 214

8 — temporal fossa 548 312 448 212

9 — anterior nasal spine 319 714 819 744

10 — body of maxilla 518 312 818 212

11 — lower jaw 514 317 914 817

12 — zygomatic bone 519 312 819 212

13 — zygomatic arch 528 317 918 917

14 — styloid process 528 917 728 918

15 — condylar process of the lower jaw 219 377 889 989

16 — mastoid 918 217 319 817

17 — external auditory meatus 528 317 918 227

18 — lambdoid suture 428 711 318 911

19 — squamous part of occipital bone 518 712 818 912

20 — superior temporal line 428 712 318 421

21 — squamous part of the temporal bone 512 821 318 921

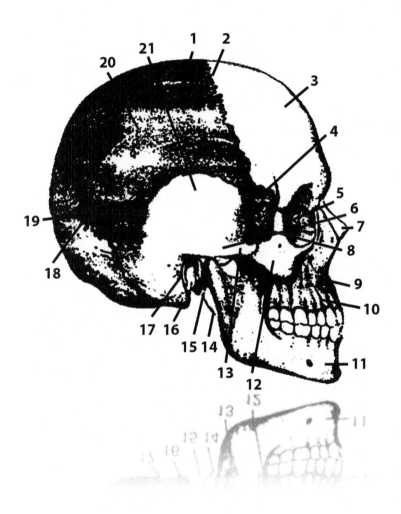

Fig. 77. The internal base of skull 519 318 418 917:

1 — orbital part of the frontal bone 998 261 378 471

2 — cockscomb 428 312 818 222

3 — cribriform lamina 428 217 328 917

4 — visual channel 555 888 918 419

5 — pituitary fossa 317 218 917 888

6 — dorsum sellae 513 988 813 488

7 — round aperture 548 321 918 489

8 — oval foramen 548 321 918 317

9 — lacerated aperture 529 317 216 489

10 — spinous aperture 528 317 918 527

11 — internal acoustic meatus 548 712 218 332

12 — jugular aperture 589 317 919 897

13 — hypoglossal canal 319 317 919 777

14 — lambdoid suture 489 312 219 812

15 — clivus 519 312 819 222

16 — sulcus of the transverse sinus 529 316 719 226

17 — internal occipital protuberance 519 317 919 227

18 — large (occipital) aperture 549 317 819 227

19 — occipital squama 529 312 819 272

20 — sulcus of sigmoid sinus 599 087 219 317

21 — pyramid (petrous) part of temporal bone 419 317 819 227

22 — squamous part of temporal bone 519 312 819 222

23 — greater wing of sphenoid bone 222 719 333 419

24 — lesser wing of sphenoid bone 213 914 817 977

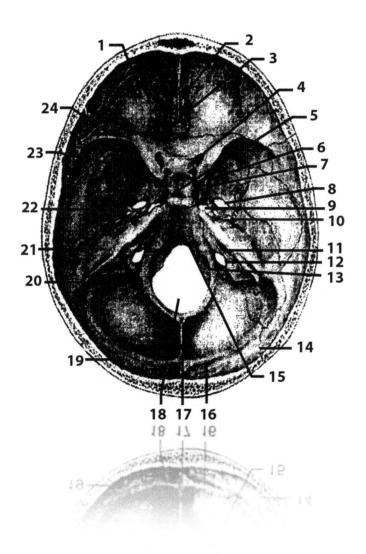

Fig. 78. Outer base of skull 894 312 918 322:

1 — palatine process of maxilla 819 312 419 222

2 — incisal aperture 498 555 978 377

3 — median palatine suture 519 312 919 222

4 — transverse palatine suture 478 217 378 227

5 — choana 529 371 999 811

6 — inferior nasal concha 519 317 519 817

7 — zygomatic arch 819 317 919 978

8 — wing of vomer 918 312 818 212

9 — pterygoid fossa 419 817 219 317

10 — lateral plate of pterygoid bone 548 321 918 221

11 — pterygoid bone 219 311 919 211

12 — oval foramen 214 715 819 315

13 — mandibular fossa 558 912 918 222

14 — styloid process 419 715 219 355

15 — external auditory meatus 914 712 814 312

16 — mastoid 548 317 918 227

17 — mastoid notch 519 312 819 221

18 — occipital condyle 514 312 788 918

19 — condylar fossa 828 213 319 712

20 — large (occipital) aperture 219 714 819 814

21 — inferior nuchal line 514 319 219 289

22 — external occipital protuberance 428 913 728 953

23 — pharyngeal tubercle 298 217 319 228

24 — condylar canal 218 317 218 227

25 — jugular foramen 891 317 919 217

26 — occipito-mastoid suture 214 312 827 488

27 — external carotic aperture 389 219 217 419

28 — stylomastoid aperture 519 317 219 227

29 — tattered hole 548 317 289 327

30 — petrotympanic fissure 219 317 418 227

31 — spinous aperture 219 317 218 227

32 — articular tubercle 288 412 298 322

33 — sphenosquamous suture 298 717 298 277

34 — pterygoid hamulus 598 328 219 830

35 — greater palatine foramen 219 498 817 312

36 — zygomaticomaxillary suture 529 312 919 812

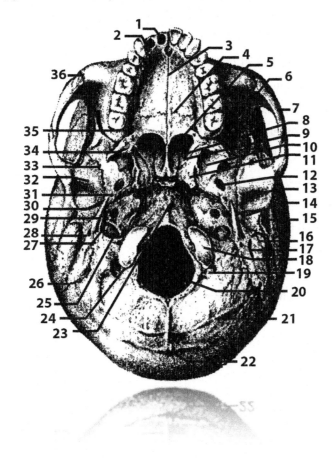

SKELETON OF LIMBS 548 212 788 272

BONES OF UPPER LIMB 971 981 319 212

Fig. 79. Right shoulder blade (rear view) 429 312 819 312:

1 — cuneate process 918 318 519 714

2 — acromion 529 319 919 712

3 — lateral angle 498 712 519 282

4 — neck of scapula 498 710 218 220

5 — lateral edge 489 770 919 220

6 — inferior corner 319 814 919 814

7 — medial edge 519 311 819 911

8 — subscapular fossa 918 712 514 317

9 — posterior surface 219 712 819 222

10 — spine of scapula 498 712 328 822

11 — supraspinatus fossa 512 488 912 988

12 — incisure of scapula 319 714 819 214

13 — superior angle 428 713 818 213

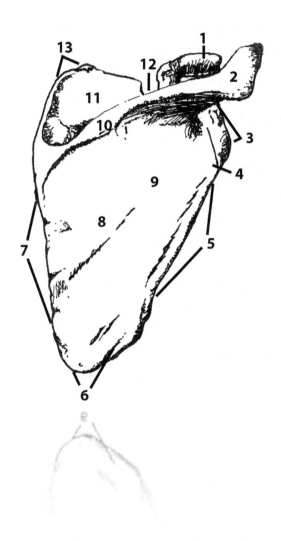

Fig. 80. Right shoulder blade (front view) 213 419 813 219:

1 — articular surface of the acromion 519 311 919 211

2 — incisure of scapula 549 811 719 311

3 — spine of scapula 519 514 318 814

4 — superior angle 519 312 819 212

5 — medial edge 598 217 317 717

6 — inferior corner 319 814 919 814

7 — lateral edge 548 312 918 212

8 — subscapular fossa 519 317 819 217

9 — costal surface 519 412 819 312

10 — neck of scapula 529 318 919 288

11 — infraglenoid tubercle 212 317 412 917

12 — lateral angle 528 318 914 818

13 — medial edge 548 912 928 312

14 — supraglenoid tubercle 488 312 818 222

15 — coracoid process 549 318 918 212

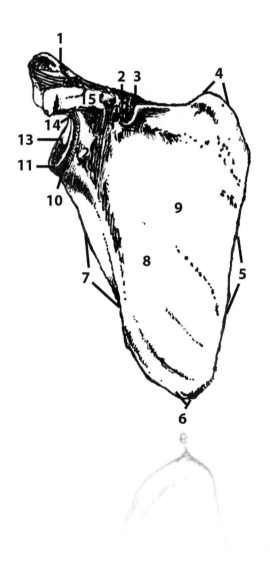

Fig. 81. Right clavicle (Bottom view) 528 312 918 222:

1 — acromial articular surface 528 314 818 214

2 — trapezoid line 428 712 928 222

3 — furrow of subclavian muscle 528 222 918 412

4 — body of clavicula 314 812 514 812

5 — sternal end 598 712 819 232

6 — sternal articular surface 548 712 918 322

7 — impression of costo-clavicular ligament 577 489 312 819

8 — cone-shaped mound 521 479 811 299

9 — acromial end 578 912 319 228

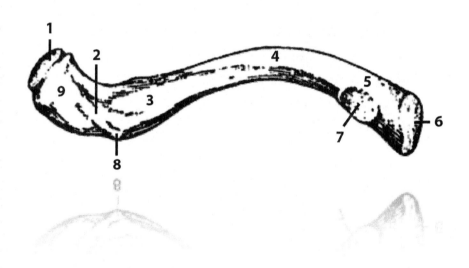

Fig. 82. Sterno-clavicular joints 512 714 312 814:

1 — costo-clavicular ligament 529 319 819 478

2 — anterior sterno-clavicular ligament 319 814 219 217

3 — midclavicular ligament 219 317 919 217

4 — articular disc 519 712 819 912

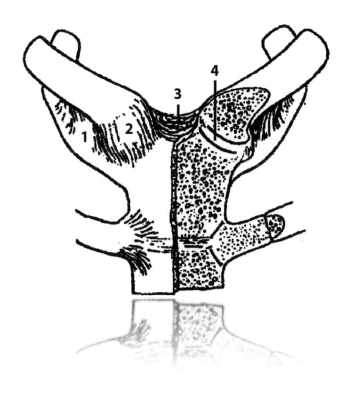

SKELETON OF FREE UPPER LIMB 219 317 918 817

Fig. 83. Right humerus (front view) 219 317 298 227:

1 — head of the humerus 219 312 819 778

2 — anatomical neck 219 312 819 887

3 — medial anterior surface 219 317 919 817

4 — medial edge 428 712 328 718

5 — condyle of the humerus 213 428 219 488

6 — medial epicondyle 219 317 819 217

7 — trochlea of the humerus 539 817 919 817

8 — head of the condyle of humerus 219 317 229 812

9 — lateral epicondyle 419 418 712 319

10 — lateral edge 513 814 713 914

11 — body of the humerus 548 912 938 817

12 — deltoid tuberosity 548 714 818 217

13 — lateral anterior surface 548 321 918 711

14 — surgical neck 542 718 312 918

15 — lesser tubercle 328 784 548 914

16 — greater tubercle 328 722 588 731

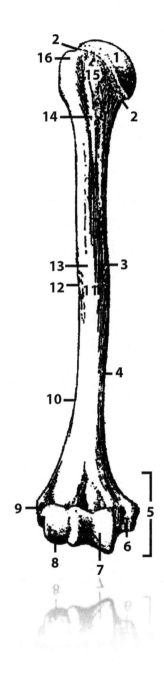

Fig. 84. Right humerus (rear view) 219 317 919 217:

1 — head of humerus 214 318 914 998

2 — anatomical neck 498 517 318 227

3 — greater tubercle 429 321 999 617

4 — surgical neck 524 319 312 218

5 — condyle of humerus 519 317 819 227

6 — lateral epicondyle 219 397 812 597

7 — fossa elbow joint 519 317 818 907

8 — trochlea of humerus 519 007 819 267

9 — furrow of ulnar nerve 298 712 319 212

10 — medial epicondyle 429 317 919 887

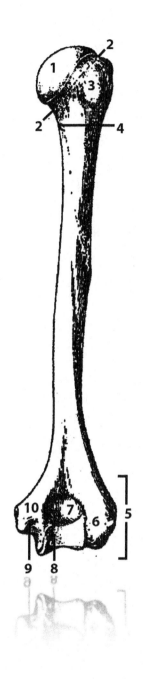

Fig. 85. Right radial and ulnar bones (front view) 598 712 498 217:

A — radial bone 531 918 898 712:

1 — head of radial bone 328 471 918 221

2 — neck of radial bone 248 312 818 222

3 — tuberosity of radius 548 712 918 272

4 — interosseous edge 548 317 918 227

5 — anterior surface 548 371 998 211

6 — anterior edge 428 317 918 917

7 — ulnar incisure 498 318 919 887

8 — carpal articular surface 319 817 919 617

9 — styloid process 514 317 914 987

10 — lateral surface 598 712 918 312

11 — body of radial bone 598 321 719 811

12 — articular circumference 549 312 919 812

B — ulna 598 712 918 222:

1 — ginglymoid incisure of 219 217 919 817

2 — coronoid process 319 374 819 814

3 — tuberosity of ulna 519 312 819 212

4 — front line 419 817 919 217

5 — body of ulna 519 321 819 221

6 — styloid process 529 326 919 726

7 — articular circumference 519 342 819 221

8 — head of ulna 548 711 919 211

9 — anterior surface 534 217 918 377

10 — interosseous edge 598 321 918 211

11 — supinator crest 498 871 218 321

12 — radial incisure 548 388 718 918

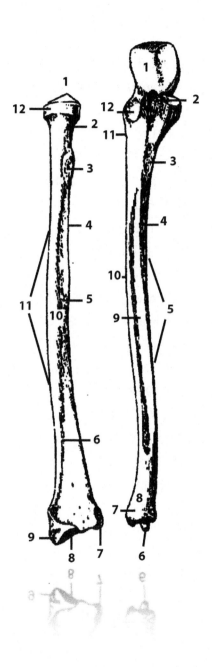

Fig. 86. Bones of the right hand
(dorsal surface) 548 722 888 222:

1 — distal phalanx 219 333 819 444

2 — middle phalanx 478 212 978 111

3 — head of phalanx 513 918 216 097

4 — phalanges (finger bones) 213 918 712 889

5 — proximal phalanx 319 712 819 222

6 — base of phalanx 519 819 312 888

7 — body of phalanx 891 319 489 519

8 — base of the metacarpal bone 519 312 919 812

9 — the third metacarpal bone 519 312 819 212

10 — body of metacarpal bone 498 712 988 318

11 — base of metacarpal bone 528 313 818 713

12 — metacarpus (I-V metacarpal bones) 598 318 488 712

13 — styloid process 528 899 319 217

14 — trapezium bone 988 713 428 755

15 — trapezoid bone 598 317 988 978

16 — capitate bone 298 317 898 007

17 — hamate bone 598 382 488 722

18 — triquetral bone 598 213 009 216

19 — pisiform bone 598 377 988 217

20 — lunate bone 598 327 918 227

21 — navicular bone 599 891 488 788

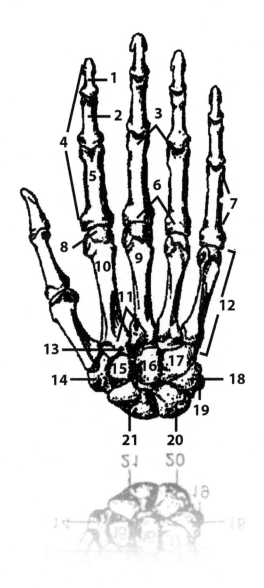

JOINTS OF UPPER LIMB 519 513 819 213

Fig. 87. Shoulder joint (longitudinal view) 219 419 213 818:
1 — tendon of the long head of biceps muscle of arm 529 321 919 478
2, 7 — articular bag 471 818 321 988
3 — acromion of scapula 519 312 948 212
4 — superior transverse ligament of scapula 519 312 919 812
5 — scapula 219 312 988 712
6 — glenoid cavity of scapula 918 317 988 817

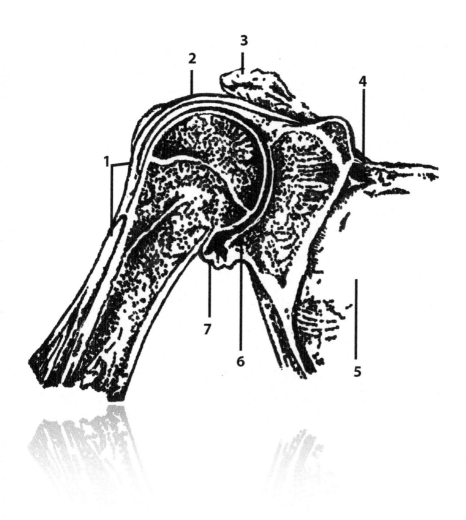

Fig. 88. Right elbow joint (front view) 598 312 419 812:

1 — humerus 918 714 988 814

2 — coronoid fossa 599 917 319 878

3 — medial epicondyle 898 321 488 712

4, 13, 14 — ligaments 519 312 819 212

5 — trochlea of humerus 599 041 319 799

6 — coronoid process 898 312 918 002

7 — tuberosity of ulnar bone 519 217 918 328

8 — ulnar bone 529 341 419 811

9 — interosseous membrane of forearm 918 312 888 512

10 — radial bone 498 712 519 322

11 — tuberosity of the radial bone 598 213 588 234

12 — tendon of biceps muscle of arm 528 377 948 724

15 — head of the humerus 548 317 489 377

16 — lateral epicondyle 219 321 891 489

17 — radial fossa 529 213 719 333

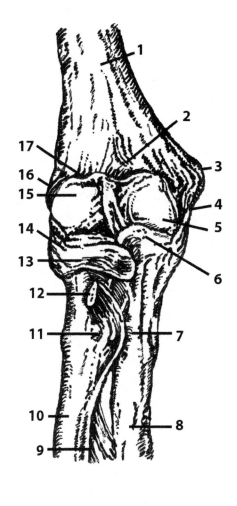

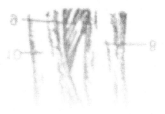

BONES OF LOWER LIMB 529 531 919 811

BELT OF LOWER LIMB 429 712 918 222

Fig. 89-A Pelvic bone; (right) 214 317 918 227:

A — view from the lateral side:

1 — iliac crest 298 327 918 887

2 — inner lip 291 398 218 612

3 — intermediate line 549 715 819 315

4 — external lip 599 422 899 322

5 — superior anterior iliac spine 529 312 919 914

6 — inferior anterior iliac spine 598 714 818 914

7 — supratrochanteric groove 594 321 714 811

8 — body of iliac bone 548 377 914 817

9 — edge of the acetabulum 519 718 918 212

10 — lunate surface 498 712 519 312

11 — fossa of acetabular cavity 548 712 918 312

12 — notch of acetabular cavity 509 714 219 314

13 — acetabulum 591 614 318 790

14 — obturator foramen 521 782 219 332

15 — ischial tuberosity 529 312 918 812

16 — ischial spine 898 918 314 517

17 — posterior gluteal line 517 318 215 428

18 — inferior posterior iliac spine 912 914 712 714

19 — superior posterior iliac spine 319 812 892 319

20 — iliac bone 519 814 319 811

21 — inferior gluteal line 519 312 891 421

22 — gluteal area 519 311 819 211

23 — wing of ilium 529 301 229 721

24 — anterior gluteal line 498 312 898 222

25 — iliac tubercle 594 312 894 222

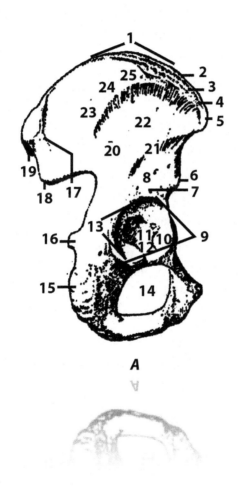

A

Fig. 89-B Pelvic bone; (right) 214 317 918 227:

B — view from the medial side:

1 — iliac crest 491 213 719 223

2 — superior posterior iliac spine 298 312 818 712

3 — sacro-pelvic surface 298 712 518 312

4 — iliac tuberosity 498 213 009 671

5 — inferior posterior iliac spine 498 319 819 007

6 — auriculate surface 931 489 219 819

7 — obturator foramen 521 798 988 122

8 — curved line 512 098 096 681

9 — inferior anterior iliac spine 319 489 091 213

10 — body of ilium 488 714 818 381

11 — iliac bone 428 713 819 223

12 — superior anterior iliac spine 219 006 789 321

13 — iliac fossa 489 091 213 719

14 — wing of ilium 519 489 389 712

15 — inner lip 528 421 389 001

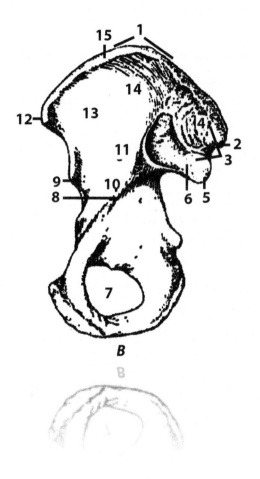

B

SKELETON OF FREE PART OF LOWER LIMB 298 321 918 557

Fig. 90. Right femoral bone (front view) 594 321 794 851:

1 — head of femoral bone 519 517 919 917

2 — fovea of the femoral bone head 319 318 919 818

3 — femoral neck 498 312 718 212

4 — intertrochanteric line 519 312 219 772

5 — lesser trochanter 918 714 518 914

6 — body of the femoral bone 598 712 918 222

7 — adductor tubercle of femur 498 312 000 612

8 — medial epicondyle 469 718 919 318

9 — medial condyle 598 317 898 617

10 — patellar surface 514 318 914 888

11 — lateral condyle 598 314 888 914

12 — lateral epicondyle 519 714 814 919

13 — greater trochanter 529 318 729 888

14 — trochanteric fossa 598 712 888 412

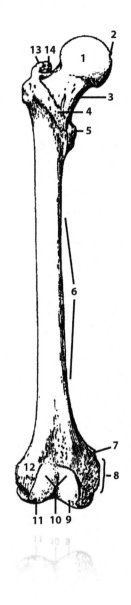

Fig. 91. Right tibial and peroneal bones (front view) 519 714 479 509:

1 — lateral condyle 519 514 319 314

2 — lateral intercondylous tubercle 539 712 819 222

3 — intercondylar eminence 548 917 328 227

4 — medial intercondylous tubercle 219 713 829 223

5 — medial condyle 394 815 519 815

6 — anterior intercondylar area 319 712 819 212

7 — articular surface of fibula head 514 317 814 227

8 — tuberosity of tibia 529 327 819 227

9 — medial surface 548 912 914 272

10 — anterior edge 428 319 819 228

11 — body of tibia 829 714 329 214

12 — medial border 314 812 914 712

13 — lateral surface 519 312 914 212

14 — medial malleolus 589 741 299 421

15 — articular surface of malleolus 528 714 328 214

16 — inferior articular surface 594 321 317 811

17 — articular surface of the fibula malleolus 598 712 918 241

18 — lateral malleolus of fibula 514 718 914 318

19 — medial surface of fibula 489 916 769 817

20 — body of fibula 538 714 918 214

21 — anterior edge of fibula 298 718 314 228

22 — lateral surface of fibula 298 317 918 227

23 — neck of fibula 238 714 214 816

24 — head of fibula 519 317 919 221

25 — apex of fibular head 518 318 918 227

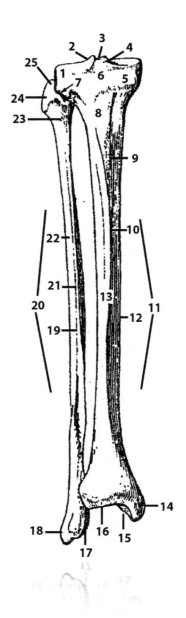

Fig. 92. Bones of the right foot (top view) 594 317 214 817:

1 — heel bone 594 312 814 712

2 — astragalus 594 317 814 227

3 — cuboid bone 598 317 998 217

4 — navicular bone 598 317 918 228

5 — cuneiform bones 284 318 914 278

6 — metatarsal (I-V) bones 918 714 888 914

7 — head of metatarsal bone 538 717 918 227

8 — finger bones (proximal; middle and distal
    phalanges) 598 317 888 999

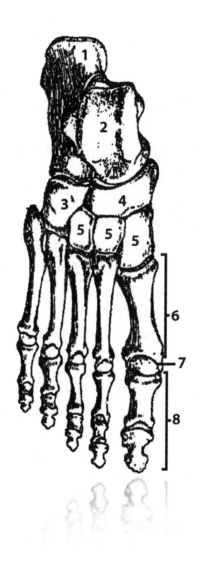

JOINTS OF LOWER LIMB 918 999 000 818

Fig. 93. Hip joint (right) 319 489 219 318:

1 — articular cartilage 219 914 319 814

2 — hip bone 519 317 819 227

3 — joint cavity 519 318 919 888

4 — ligament of femoral bone head 548 317 228 917

5 — transverse ligament of acetabulum 514 318 814 228

6 — joint capsule 987 421 328 921

7 — ischial tuberosity 598 714 318 227

8 — circular area 598 712 998 212

9 — acetabular lip 219 317 559 417

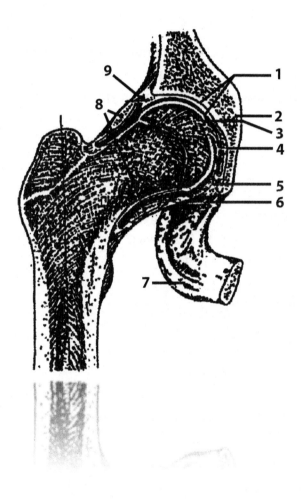

Fig. 94. Knee joint 419 718 214 328:

1 — femoral bone 219 317 919 817

2 — tibial collateral ligament 519 312 819 272

3 — medial condyle 498 712 919 812

4 — posterior cruciate ligament 419 321 819 221

5 — anterior cruciate ligament 219 314 919 814

6 — medial meniscus 519 312 819 212

7 — tibia 521 918 519 818

8 — patellar tendon 594 312 894 882

9 — patella 548 316 918 716

10 — fibula bone 988 712 819 212

11 — fibula collateral ligament 529 317 889 227

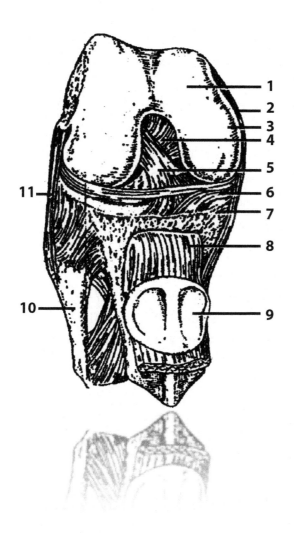

1
2
3
4
5
6
7
8
9
10
11

Fig. 95. Joints and ligaments of right foot 419 417 819 817:

1 — tibia 529 321 819 221

2 — cavity ankle 429 327 919 877

3, 7, 12, 13, 16, 18, 19, 20, 21, 23 — ligaments; strengthening
joints 219 317 819 227

4 — transverse tarsal joint 391 819 291 919

5 — navicular bone 419 891 599 211

6 — cuneonavicular articulation 514 387 914 327

8, 9, 10 — cuneiform bones 519 712 819 222

11 — tarsometatarsal joints 519 518 919 818

14 — interphalangeal joints 514 217 914 317

15 — metatarsal-phalanx joint (V) 594 312 814 212

17 — cuboid bone 394 812 944 212

22 — subtalar joint 594 317 814 217

24 — fibula 598 317 919 817

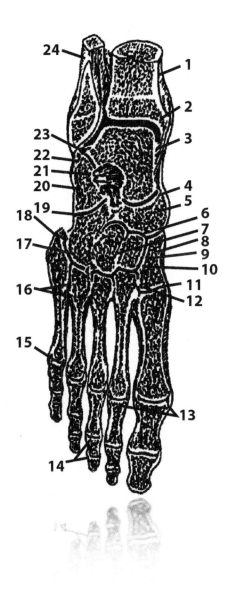

MUSCLE SYSTEM 214 712 314 222

Fig. 96. Numerical concentrations
on shape of muscles 898 811 919 218:

A — fusiform 319 241 809 217

B — biceps muscle 914 312 219 312

C — digastric muscle 214 318 914 718

D — muscle with tendinous intersections 519 317 914 817

E — pinnate muscle 498 712 319 212

F — semipenniform muscle 519 314 219 814

1 — muscle belly 594 312 814 212

2, 3 — muscle tendons 598 317 918 227

4 — tendinous intersection 519 817 919 227

5 — intermediate tendon 319 919 819 318

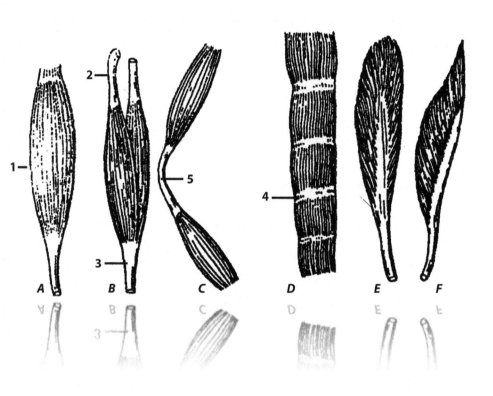

Concentration on numbers restoring form of matter allow to apply the appropriate spiritual state to such concentrations to recover the form of certain organs and the whole organism.

MUSCLES AND FASCIA OF TORSO 514 312 814 212

Fig. 97. Superficial muscles of the back 819 314 914 812:

1 — Belt muscle of the head 214 312 814 212

2 — muscle lifting scapula 214 317 914 717

3 — lesser rhomboid muscle 519 312 819 212

4 — large rhomboid muscle 219 317 919 817

5 — inferior posterior notched muscle 549 317 919 817

6 — lumbar-thoracic fascia 529 317 919 817

7 — latissimus muscle of back 429 318 829 998

8 — trapezius muscle 421 317 921 817

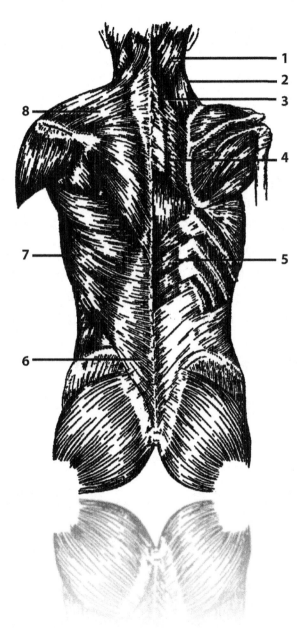

Fig. 98. Suboccipital muscles 531 814 212 814:

1 — interspinous muscles of neck 498 712 818 212

2 — intertransverse muscles 519 314 819 312

3 — inferior oblique muscle of head 218 317 918 227

4 — superior oblique muscle of head 218 417 918 817

5 — Large posterior rectus of head 419 317 819 227

6 — lesser posterior rectus of head 219 817 819 227

BACK FASCIITIS 214 718 314 888

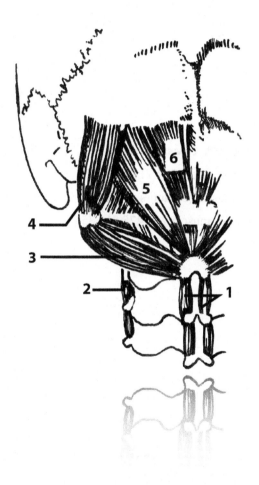

Fig. 99. Chest muscles 498 712 818 212:

1 — major pectoral muscle 214 718 918 228

2 — minor chest muscle (contours of muscle) 219 312 819 242

3 — serratus anterior muscle 219 475 819 355

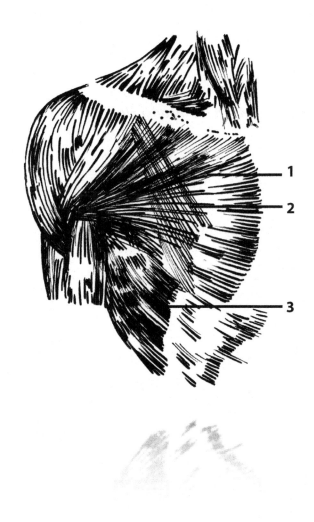

1

2

3

Fig. 100. Aperture (bottom view) 219 289 228 317:

1 — sternal part of diaphragm 519 517 819 217

2, 10 — costal part of diaphragm 214 312 489 212

3 — tendinous center 519 317 919 217

4 — aperture for the inferior vena cava 519 518 919 218

5 — hole for esophagus 528 317 918 227

6 — aperture for aorta 548 312 918 227

7, 8, 9 — feet of lumbar part of diaphragm 549 316 860 219

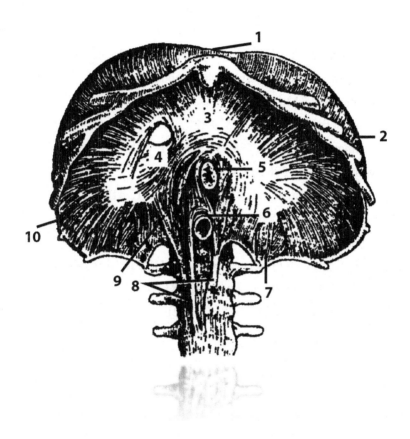

Fig. 101. Abdominal muscles 517 318 917 918:

1 — aponeurosis of the external oblique abdominal
muscles 914 312 814 212

2 — rectus abdominis 598 712 319 217

3 — tendinous intersection 528 714 328 917

4 — internal oblique 398 217 818 417

5 — external oblique muscle of abdomen 529 312 419 272

6 — pyramidal muscle 598 742 218 228

7, 8 — posterior wall of the rectus sheath 213 019 514 219

9 — aponeurosis of transversus abdominis 418 714 918 444

10 — transversus abdominis muscle 555 813 915 513

11 — abdomen white line 319 481 219 321

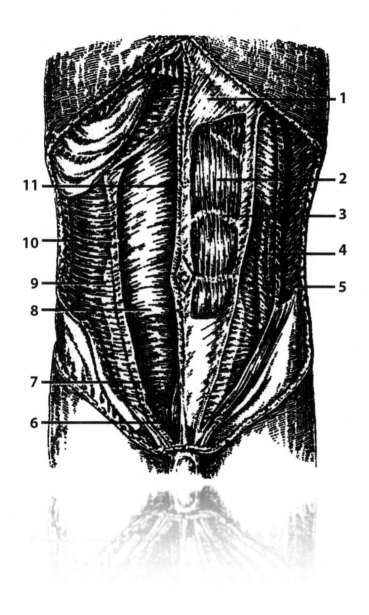

MUSCLES AND FASCIA OF HEAD AND NECK 219 214 419 314

Fig. 102. Superficial facial muscles of head 219 317 914 817:

1 — epicranial aponeurosis 314 812 914 212

2 — occipito-frontal muscle 009 812 214 312

3, 6, 7 — circular muscle of eye 214 317 914 217

4 — procerus muscle 829 312 714 712

5 — circular muscle of mouth 548 321 818 221

8 — temporo-parietal muscle 409 641 219 741

9 — anterior auricular muscle 519 312 518 222

10 — posterior auricular muscle 548 314 214 317

11 — occipito-frontal muscle 518 714 318 214

12 — upper auricular muscle 519 812 919 912

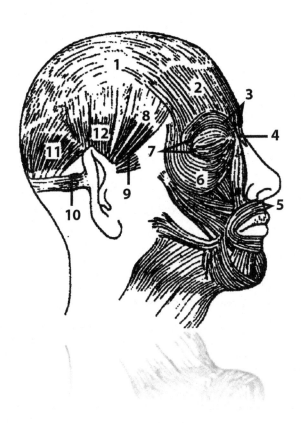

Fig. 103. Facial muscles (front view) 548 321 918 221:

1 — muscle lifting the corner of the mouth 598 712 918 242

2 — buccal muscle 549 317 849 217

3 — masticatory muscle 598 712 918 212

4 — mentalis 314 312 814 212

5 — transversus chin muscle 519 712 819 212

6 — platysma 518 317 918 227

7 — muscles lowering bottom lip 521 319 221 919

8 — muscles driving the angle of the mouth 518 519 318 919

9 — risorius muscle 418 716 818 999

10 — zygomaticus major muscle 548 712 998 218

11 — minor zygomatic muscle 598 217 918 227

12 — the muscle lifting the upper lip 319 817 219 227

13 — muscle lifting the upper lip and nose wing 419 227 299 327

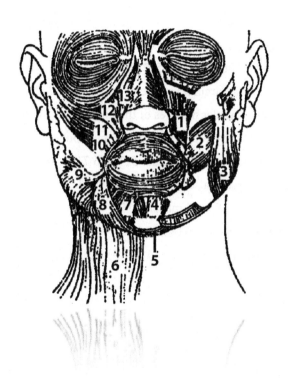

Fig. 104. Deep facial muscles 328 721 428 919:

1 — muscle wrinkling eyebrow 512 428 912 728

2 — lacrimal part of circular muscle of the eye 319 742 819 222

3 — edge part of circular muscles of the mouth 548 232 619 722

4 — labial part of the circular muscles of the mouth 428 713 918 523

5 — muscles lowering nasal septum 521 216 719 226

6 — alar part of nasal muscles 428 921 321 481

7 — transverse part of nasal muscle 219 317 819 228

8 — nasal muscle 498 712 518 232

9 — muscle lowering eyebrow 514 217 914 217

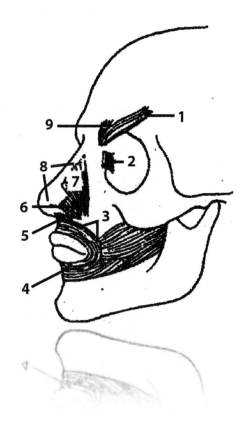

MASTICATORY MUSCLES 519 314 819 214

Fig. 105. Masticatory muscles 519 314 819 214:

1 — temporalis muscle 218 317 918 217

2 — lateral pterygoid 219 214 319 214

3 — medial pterygoid 819 912 314 272

4 — buccal muscle 518 222 319 272

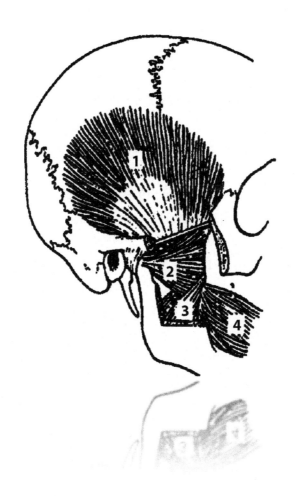

FASCIA OF HEAD 519 718 218 314

Fig. 106. Fascia of head 519 718 218 314:

1 — temporal fascia 319 814 919 214

2 — deep layer of temporal fascia 519 312 919 212

3 — parotid fascia 519 814 719 314

4 — chewing fascia 514 312 814 212

5 — platysma 538 312 918 712

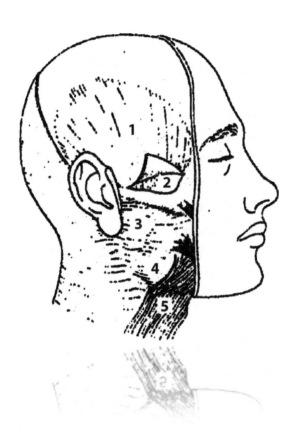

NECK MUSCLES 548 007 998 227

Fig. 107. Muscles of head and neck
(right side and bottom view) 528 342 918 712:

1 — masseter 428 317 918 227

2 — deep part of masseter 574 321 914 211

3 — superficial part of masseter 584 312 984 212

4 — bucco-pharyngeal fascia 217 317 519 715

5 — sternocleidomastoid muscle 548 712 218 312

6 — digastric 214 318 914 718

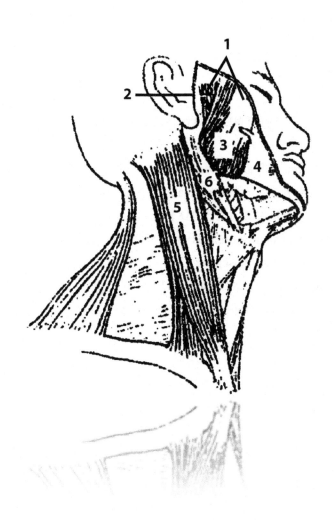

DEEP NECK MUSCLES 819 341 919 841

Fig. 108. Deep muscles of neck 819 341 919 841:

1 — anterior rectus muscle of head 214 712 814 312

2 — long muscle of neck 213 418 913 818

3 — anterior scalene muscle 319 812 919 212

4 — middle scalene muscle 489 316 718 916

5 — long muscle of head 519 817 319 817

6 — lateral rectus muscle of head 519 314 819 214

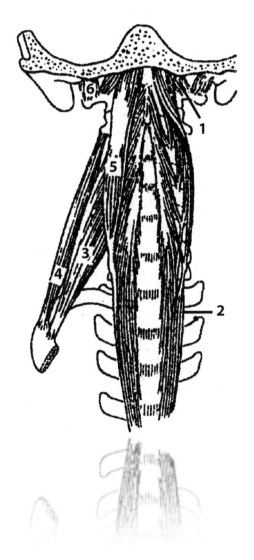

MUSCLES AND FASCIA OF
UPPER EXTREMITY 219 314 819 914

Fig. 109. Girdle muscles and
shoulder (front view) 498 711 598 321:

1 — subscapularis muscle 519 312 219 282

2 — large circular muscle 459 321 989 721

3 — coracoid-shoulder muscle 219 371 419 871

4 — coracobrachial muscle 419 812 599 322

5, 10 — shoulder muscle 548 321 718 211

6 — humeral head of round pronator 598 317 819 217

7 — round pronator 519 314 819 214

8 — ulnar head of round pronator 919 814 319 214

9 — aponeurosis biceps muscle of arm 428 312 818 512

11 — long head of biceps 519 817 919 017

12 — short head of biceps 584 712 584 389

13 — biceps brachii 549 817 319 217

14 — intertubercular tendon sheath of long head of
biceps 214 987 914 317

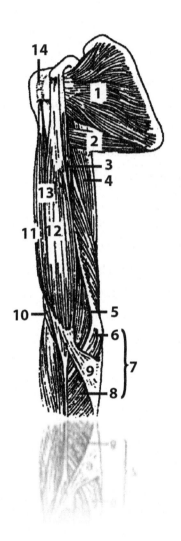

Fig. 110. Muscles of girdle of superior
extremity and arm (rear view) 519 312 819 289:

1 — supraspinatus 312 214 812 514

2 — infraspinatus muscle 598 712 918 222

3 — small circular muscle 555 333 918 433

4 — deltoid 598 371 888 911

5 — lateral head of triceps brachii 598 909 913 718

6 — triceps brachii 419 812 599 322

7, 9 — medial head of triceps brachii 529 382 728 814

8 — anconeus 517 214 917 814

10 — long head of triceps brachii 512 718 912 229

11 — large circular muscle 919 813 914 312

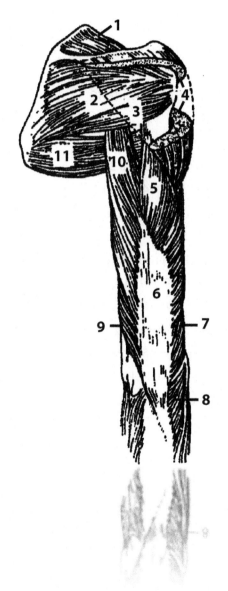

Fig. 111. Forearm muscles (front group) 519 317 819 217:

A — surface:

1 — bicipital aponeurosis 514 312 814 712

2 — biceps 319 812 919 912

3 — round pronator 419 841 899 541

4 — long palmar muscle 498 715 318 225

5 — ulnar flexor of wrist 519 314 819 214

6 — humeroulnar head of superficial flexor digitorum
    longus 513 819 913 514

7 — superficial flexors 319 811 919 891

8 — short palmar muscle 598 319 719 818

9 — square pronator 519 317 918 517

10 — radial head superficial flexor digitorum 598 317 588 817

11 — long radial wrist extensor 598 214 319 814

12 — radial wrist flexor 511 408 219 319

13 — brachioradialis muscle 914 312 814 212

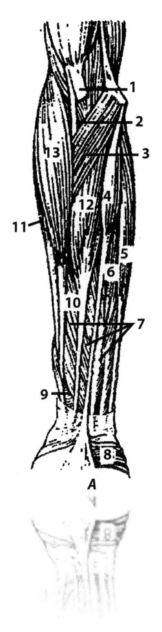

A

Fig. 112. Right hand muscles (front view) 214 717 814 327:

1 — flexor retinaculum 519 321 019 614

2 — muscle abductor of little finger 318 912 818 006

3 — short flexor of little finger 519 388 498 514

4 — deep flexor tendons of fingers 588 317 918 777

5 — opposer muscle of little finger 988 888 314 007

6 — lumbrical muscles 568 721 328 521

7 — tendons of superficial flexor of fingers 598 712 899 422

8 — adductor muscle of thumb 599 712 899 329

9 — long flexor tendon of thumb 548 916 379 816

10 — short flexor of thumb 898 317 879 917

11 — short abductor muscle of thumb 389 671 899 211

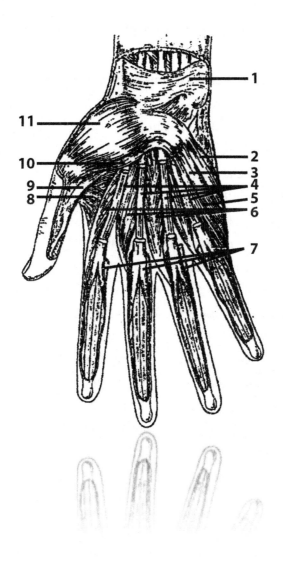

LOWER EXTREMITY MUSCLES 514 311 914 527

PELVIC MUSCLES 298 317 919 817

Fig. 113-A Muscles of lower extremity 528 317 918 787:

A — Front View:

1 — iliopsoas muscle 319 311 919 811

2 — pectineal muscle 519 712 918 412

3 — adductor longus 519 312 819 712

4 — thin muscle 319 042 219 822

5 — sartorius muscle 899 389 919 388

6 — medial vastus muscle 988 091 891 491

7 — quadriceps tendon muscle 514 517 814 317

8 — patellar tendon 519 514 319 814

9 — gastrocnemius muscle 589 319 814 228

10 — salens muscle 498 513 818 933

11 — long extensor digitorum 318 512 818 064

12 — long peroneal muscle 528 426 918 726

13 — anterior tibial muscle 548 717 318 917

14 — vastus lateralis muscle 548 964 328 744

15 — rectus femoris 589 371 841 218

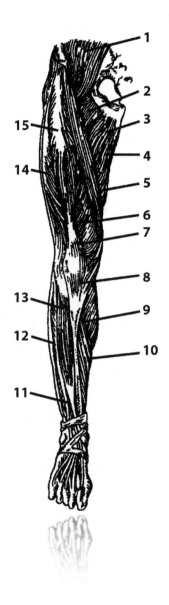

Fig. 113-B Muscles of lower extremity 528 317 918 787:

B — rear view:

1 — gluteus maximus muscle 514 317 814 227

2 — ilio-tibial tract (part of the fascia lata) 219 371 819 511

3 — biceps femoris 598 617 329 817

4 — gastrocnemius muscle 589 319 814 228

5 — achilles tendon 598 317 418 917

6 — semimembranous muscle 388 427 918 227

7 — semitendinosus muscle 549 381 714 817

MUSCLES OF FREE PART OF LOWER LIMB 319 715 819 555

LEG MUSCLES 329 481 918 511

FOOT MUSCLES 519 371 819 511

FASCIA OF LOWER LIMB 529 377 429 879

CRURAL FASCIA 539 427 819 677

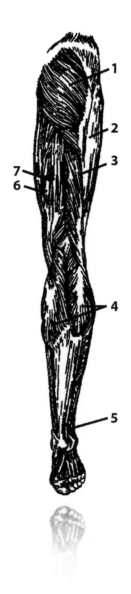

INTERNAL ORGANS 523 000 898 111

DIGESTIVE SYSTEM 541 928 741 588

Fig. 114. Digestive tract 514 388 914 888:

1 — pharynx 519 987 319 427

2 — esophagus 598 381 698 711

3 — stomach 898 898 478 213

4 — place where the stomach transites into duodenum 598 513 998 719

5 — place where the duodenum transites into jejunum 214 511 819 311

6 — jejunum 548 714 318 215

7 — descending colon 248 389 428 999

8 — sigmoid colon 319 812 519 427

9 — rectum 598 714 898 314

10 — appendix 529 317 899 228

11 — ileum 394 897 594 377

12 — cecum 519 489 319 788

13 — ascending colon 599 213 988 713

14 — duodenum 589 608 488 914

BUCCAL CAVITY 891 000 499 887

ORAL GLANDS 319 841 519 811

PHARYNX 398 715 918 455

ESOPHAGUS 214 317 988 578

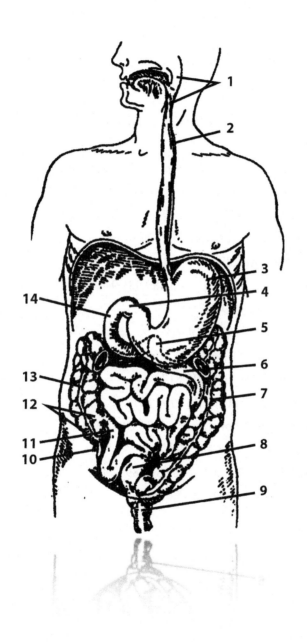

1

2

3

4

5

6

7

8

9

10

11

12

13

14

STOMACH 898 898 478 213

Fig. 115. Stomach 898 898 478 213:

1 — the bottom of stomach 898 319 899 214

2 — anterior wall 514 878 917 887

3 — folds of stomach 598 317 918 527

4 — body of stomach 889 919 389 418

5 — greater curvature of stomach 489 981 948 513

6 — pyloric canal 518 917 319 877

7 — pyloric cave 548 711 919 411

8 — pyloric antrum 591 488 791 888

9 — corner notch 596 317 549 817

10 — stomach channel 599 481 799 811

11 — small curvature of stomach 418 728 319 348

12 — cardiac orifice 528 481 798 711

13 — cardiac part of stomach 521 316 891 714

14 — cardial notch 517 916 815 322

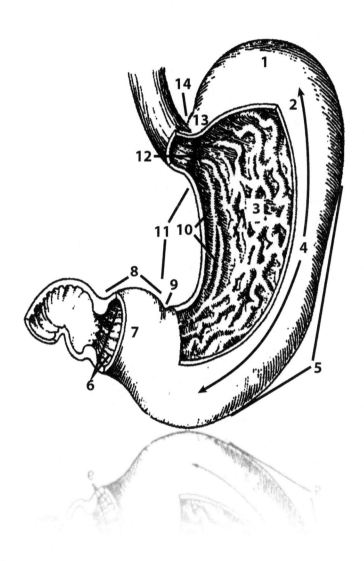

Fig. 116. Muscular layer of stomach 4981 516 018 329:

1, 8 — longitudinal layer 599 891 799 811

2 — oblique fibers 534 981 814 917

3, 4 — circular layer 599 317 819 417

5 — pylorus 598 421 918 511

6 — hole pylorus 598 714 818 314

7 — pyloric sphincter 598 714 918 324

9 — muscular layer 584 321 844 711

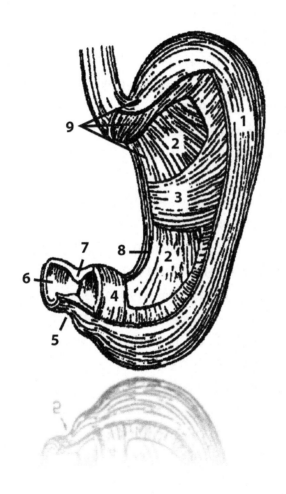

SMALL INTESTINE 528 317 428 717

LIVER, DUODENUM, PANCREAS 219 214 319 714

Fig. 117. Liver, duodenum, pancreas 219 214 319 714:

1 — left triangular ligament 519 617 919 817

2 — left lobe of liver 988 411 218 217

3 — crescent ligament (liver) 214 311 714 811

4 — common hepatic duct 914 311 814 019

5 — pancreas 589 317 919 877

6 — common bile duct 599 381 989 391

7 — tail of pancreas 898 429 719 482

8 — pancreatic duct 599 316 739 928

9 — duodenal skinny-bending 214 279 881 319

10 — jejunum 519 718 919 818

11 — ascending part of duodenum 591 477 391 817

12 — head of pancreas 319 487 914 917

13 — horizontal part of duodenum 519 314 819 414

14 — descending part of duodenum 019 819 319 417

15 — superior part of duodenum 519 811 919 311

16 — cystic duct 599 811 919 891

17 — gall bladder 918 712 418 912

18 — right triangular ligament 588 918 319 819

19 — coronary ligament 514 312 914 812

20 — right lobe of liver 519 317 914 817

LARGE INTESTINE 591 488 898 217

ABDOMEN AND PERITONEUM 598 123 098 719

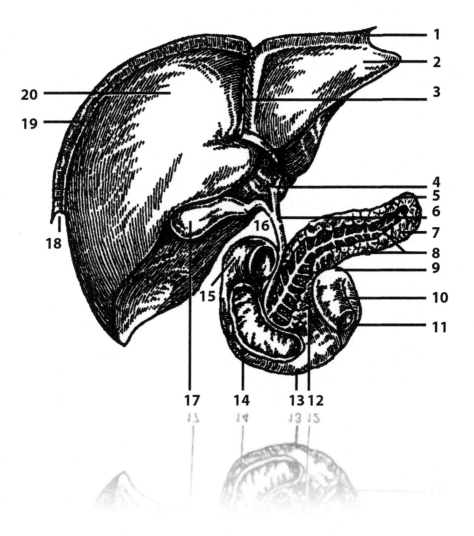

20
19
18

1
2
3
4
5
6
7
8
9
10
11

16
15
17 14 13 12

RESPIRATORY SYSTEM 598 788 428 317

NASAL CAVITY 214 711 898 219

LARYNX 291 891 419 391

LARYNGEAL CARTILAGES 529 319 489 518
LARYNX MUSCLES 594 318 719 214
LARYNX CAVITY 581 398 421 898

Fig. 118. Cavity of larynx (front view) 519 314 819 217:

1 — epiglottis 214 317 814 817

2 — epiglottic tubercle 219 329 814 718

3 — vestibule of larynx 519 481 299 811

4 — fold vestibule 599 016 719 317

5 — laryngeal ventricle 528 391 919 811

6 — vocal fold 598 718 319 421

7 — thyroid cartilage 588 421 388 711

8 — glottis 528 742 318 014

9 — infraglottic cavity 514 781 910 094

10 — tracheal cavity 298 719 488 919

11 — cricoid 584 317 589 307

12 — lateral cricoarytenoid 219 387 919 227

13 — voice muscle 594 817 914 919

14 — cricoarytenoid muscle 513 819 014 912

15 — fissure vestibule 598 741 998 328

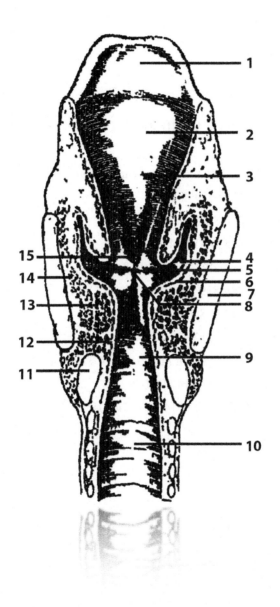

TRACHEA AND BRONCHI 428 714 008 914

Fig. 119. Trachea, bronchi and lungs 891 321 511 981:

1 — trachea 429 318 919 888

2 — apex of lung 598 712 918 212

3 — superior lobe 529 312 547 399

4a — oblique fissure 498 712 818 918

4b — horizontal slit 819 321 918 898

5 — lower lobe 214 318 718 912

6 — medial lobe 519 812 919 422

7 — cardiac notch of the left lung 519 514 319 814

8 — main bronchus 819 314 899 049

9 — bifurcation of trachea 514 518 314 818

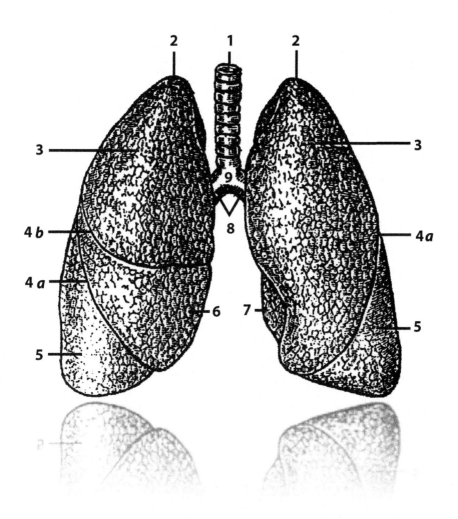

LUNGS 519 418 319 818

Fig. 120. Lung segments:

A — front view

B — rear view

C — right lung (side view)

D — left lung (side view)

1 — Segment 914 818 312 898

2 — Segment 319 814 919 914

3 — Segment 219 318 919 818

4 — Segment 519 319 818 214

5 — Segment 918 319 819 212

6 — Segment 314 819 888 915

7 — Segment 219 319 812 794

8 — Segment 319 419 898 912

9 — Segment 319 892 219 844

10 — Segment 319 488 988 210

PLEURA AND MEDIASTINUM 898 315 428 188

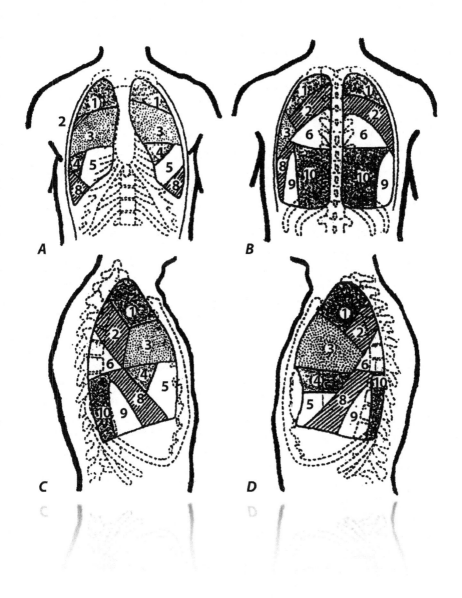

A

B

C

D

UROGENITAL APPARATUS
898 398 412 842

KIDNEY 289 391 814 216

Fig. 121. Right kidney (front view) 289 391 814 216:

1 — cortical substance 912 898 949 319

2 — medullary substance 598 716 399 008

3 — renal papillae 519 377 918 227

4 — renal poles 594 312 898 714

5 — fibrous capsule 980 841 218 329

6 — small renal calices 589 326 799 816

7 — ureter 498 712 989 322

8 — large calyx 989 217 519 487

9 — renal pelvis 928 899 499 711

10 — Renal vein 518 914 319 528

11 — renal artery 198 711 298 241

12 — renal pyramid 539 871 491 001

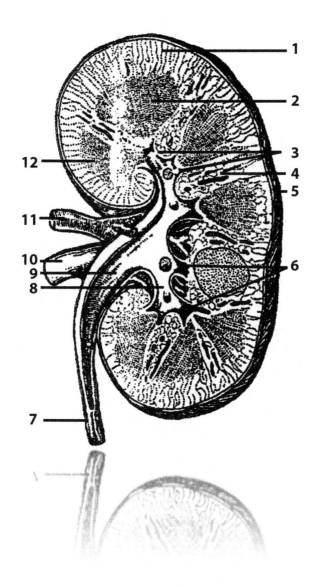

Fig. 122. Structure and blood supply of nephron:

1 — distal convoluted tubule 814 988 719 081

2 — network of capillaries 214 718 918 317

3 — collecting ducts 548 219 317 917

4 — movement of urine to the renal pelvis 298 017 498 498

5 — loop of Henle 518 319 888 910

6 — renal artery 541 890 719 019

7 — Renal vein 519 017 312 898

8 — proximal convoluted tubule 571 898 714 557

9 — bringing arterioles 889 014 219 893

10 — efferent arterioles 890 014 318 714

11 — renal glomerulus 519 891 249 318

12 — venule 213 984 791 248

13 — Bowman's capsule 298 788 489 791

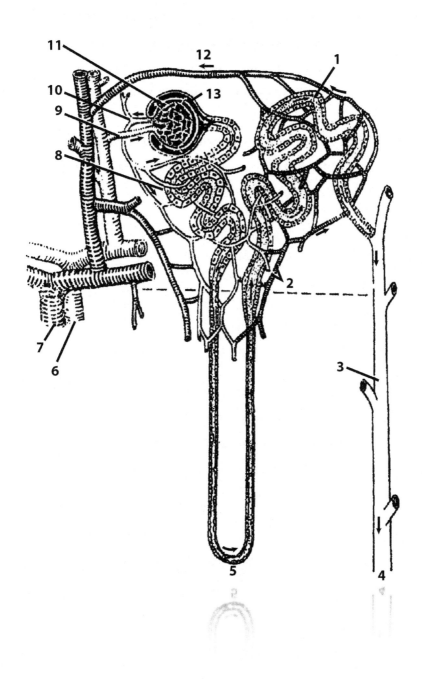

MALE GENITALIA 519 007 898 367
URETER 214 312 810 008
URINARY BLADDER 219 389 998 419
URETHRA 329 487 948 216

Fig. 123. Internal and external male genitalia:

1 — bladder 219 389 998 419

2 — seminal vesicle 519 317 898 487

3 — ejaculatory ducts 591 488 011 228

4 — membranous part of urethra 319 487 919 008

5 — crus of penis 819 317 919 847

6 — bulb of penis 528 719 048 317

7 — deferent duct 398 755 819 455

8 — spongy body 398 787 914 321

9 — cavernous body 598 721 598 311

10 — epididymis 519 488 299 318

11 — efferent tubules 548 371 818 211

12 — testicular mesh 938 729 488 219

13 — straight seminiferous tubules 419 871 989 311

14 — convoluted seminiferous tubules 498 712 819 212

15 — albuginea 319 817 919 217

16 — inferior part of deferent duct 519 891 499 217

17 — balanus 528 714 314 712

18 — bulbourethral gland 519 712 419 812

19 — prostate gland 498 714 918 214

20 — ampulla of deferent duct 418 918 971 998

21 — ureter 214 312 810 008

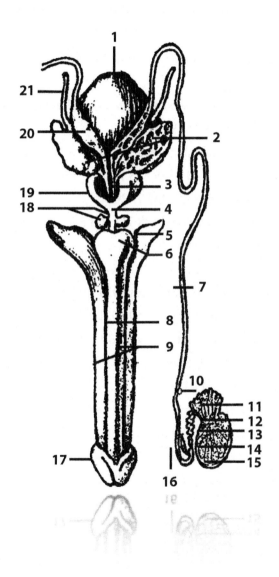

FEMALE GENITALIA 519 814 089 319

INTERNAL FEMALE GENITALIA 419 219 808 319

Fig. 124. Female external genitalia 519 319 818 678:

1 — pubis 519 317 898 498

2 — anterior commissure of lips 591 489 719 328

3 — clitoral foreskin 419 319 898 987

4 — glans of clitoris 980 409 501 201

5 — large lips of pudendum 598 711 008 512

6 — lacunar ducts 598 641 788 910

7 — small lips of pudendum 319 016 789 498

8 — large gland duct vestibule 889 014 317 489

9 — frenulum of pudendal lips 598 021 318 714

10 — posterior commissure of lips 539 421 819 317

11 — anus 589 317 418 917

12 — crotch 398 711 419 411

13 — fossa of vestibule 589 471 219 889

14 — hymen 529 314 789 064

15 — opening of vagina 591 472 918 223

16 — vestibule of vagina 888 017 989 117

17 — external urethral opening 498 663 219 773

18 — clitoris frenulum 398 421 891 871

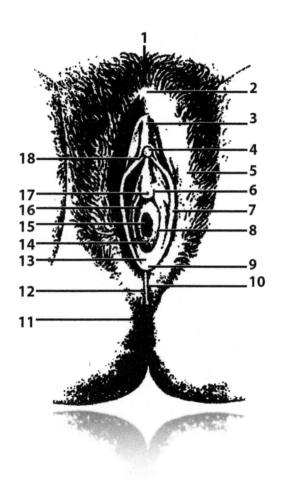

ENDOCRINE GLANDS 889 314 219 798

It is possible to perform numerical concentrations on endocrine glands by areas of their location sequentially focusing on the numbers corresponding to the endocrine glands 889 314 219 798 and on the number of organs in the area of which endocrine glands are located. This method can be applied in principle of recovering by the numerical concentrations which, along with the restoration of the chosen fabrics is appropriate for restoration of the surrounding tissue of the area. Numerical series of endocrine glands regulation 519 317 219 416 can be used to accelerate the recovery of matter.

HYPOPHYSITIS AND EPIPHYSIS 214 318 908 210
HYPOPHYSITIS 317 218 219 819

Fig. 125. Location of endocrine glands of man:

1 — cerebral hemisphere 819 917 819 319

2 — nucleus of hypothalamus 890 498 319 718

3 — hypophysis 317 218 219 819

4 — thyroid 829 319 409 819

5 — trachea 429 318 919 888

6 — lung 519 418 319 818

7 — pericardium 989 387 988 878

8 — adrenal medulla 549 378 918 268

9 — cortical substance (cortex) of adrenal gland 912 898 949 319

10 — kidney 289 391 814 216

11 — aorta 398 071 890 498

12 — bladder 219 389 998 419

13 — testicle 298 017 319 487

14 — inferior hollow vein 549 671 919 871

15 — aortic paraganglia 591 488 018 713

16 — pancreas 589 317 919 877

17 — adrenal 891 418 712 319

18 — liver 219 712 919 222

19 — thymus gland (thymus) 481 914 319 814

20 — parathyroid gland 219 319 895 219

21 — carotid body 549 641 898 017

22 — cerebellum 828 219 328 299

23 — pineal gland (epiphysis) 519 317 819 217

24 — corpus callosum 498 712 328 071

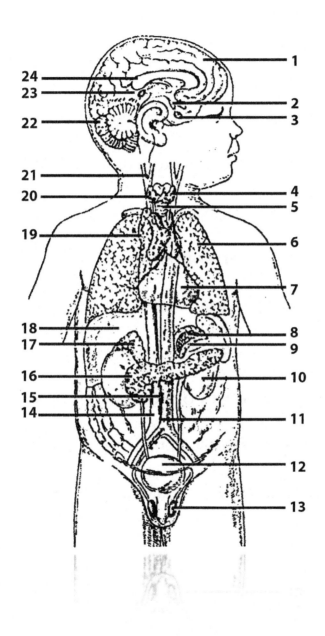

1

24
23

2
3

22

21
20

4
5

19

6

7

18
17

8
9

16

10

15
14

11

12

13

PINEAL GLAND, OR EPIPHYSIS 519 317 819 217

THYROID AND PARATHYROID GLANDS 219 318 219 471

THYMUS 481 914 319 814

THYROID 829 319 409 819

PARATHYROID GLANDS 219 319 895 219

SUPRARENAL 891 418 712 319

ENDOCRINE PART OF PANCREAS 918 712 818 229

ENDOCRINE PART OF SEXUAL GLANDS 519 318 914 019

REGULATION OF ENDOCRINE GLANDS 519 317 219 416

CARDIOVASCULAR SYSTEM
214 700 819 891

ARTERIES, VEINS AND CAPILLARIES 219 387 919 887

HEART 918 749 328 081

Fig. 126. Heart (front view) 918 749 328 081:

1 — aorta 319 498 017 819

2 — brachiocephalic trunk 998 301 248 227

3 — left common carotid artery 428 712 488 913

4 — left subclavian artery 429 387 219 377

5 — arterial ligament 214 317 814 227

6 — pulmonary trunk 519 421 819 221

7 — left ear 519 318 219 481

8, 15 — coronary sulcus 519 312 814 829

9 — left ventricle 589 348 914 918

10 — apex of the heart 519 421 899 321

11 — notch of heart apex 528 944 988 714

12 — sternocostal (front) surface of heart 519 317 988 547

13 — right ventricle 598 371 988 011

14 — anterior interventricular sulcus 909 817 398 787

16 — right ear 598 714 321 898

17 — superior hollow vein 398 712 988 012

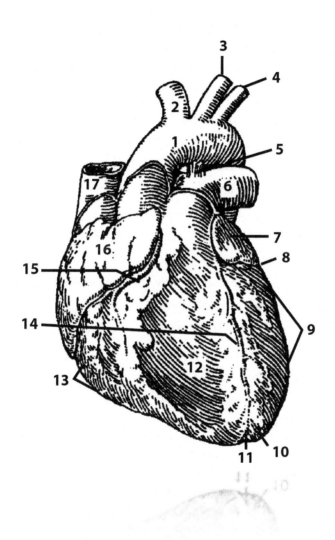

VESSELS OF PULMONARY CIRCULATION 898 714 988 569

PULMONARY VEINS 598 413 988 597

VESSELS OF GREATER CIRCULATION 598 716 588 317

AORTIC ARCH BRANCHES 298 714 319 814

Fig. 127. Heart (opened) 918 749 328 081:

1 — semilunar cusps of aortic valve 591 487 919 877

2 — pulmonary veins 309 428 519 421

3 — left atrium 518 712 314 887

4, 9 — coronary arteries 519 817 319 487

5 — left atrioventricular (mitral) valve (bicuspid valve) 598 517 818 617

6 — papillary muscles 598 717 918 317

7 — right ventricle 598 720 898 470

8 — right atrioventricular (tricuspid) valve 389 412 819 322

10 — pulmonary trunk 288 418 891 008

11 — superior hollow vein 519 312 489 098

12 — aorta 398 071 890 498

CARDIAC CONDUCTION SYSTEM 989 808 884 318

BLOOD SUPPLY AND INNERVATION
OF HEART 891 318 910 488

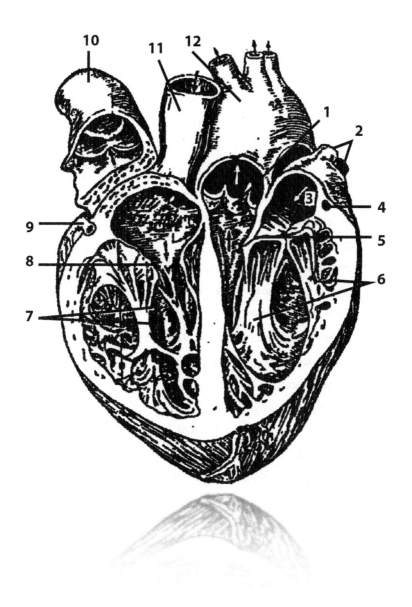

Fig. 128. Arteries of head and neck
(right side view) 518 422 819 312:

1 — dorsal nasal artery 398 718 989 061

2 — infraorbital artery 898 048 319 061

3 — angular artery 288 919 069 789

4 — superior lip artery 598 712 819 328

5 — inferior labial artery 219 318 488 519

6 — submental artery 219 319 489 555

7 — facial artery 219 061 234 890

8 — lingual artery 498 519 401 209

9 — superior thyroid artery 519 513 719 313

10 — common carotid artery 894 317 212 847

11 — inferior thyroid artery 518 377 918 478

12 — surface cervical artery 214 381 918 918

13 — thyrocervical trunk 519 317 919 288

14 — subclavian artery 594 712 819 017

15 — suprascapular artery 529 317 419 817

16 — transverse cervical artery 519 894 512 319

17 — internal carotid artery 298 012 301 914

18 — superficial temporal artery 519 016 319 417

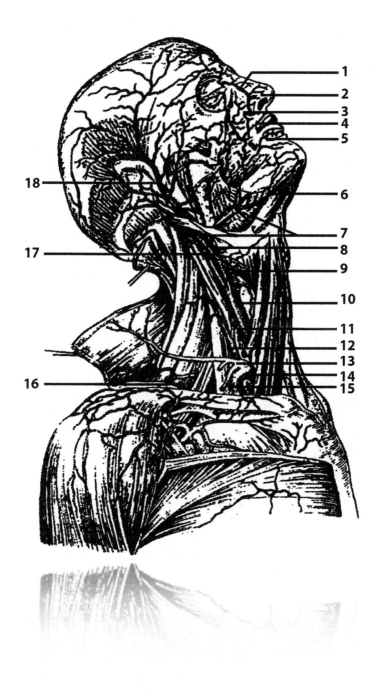

1
2
3
4
5
6
7
8
9
10
11
12
13
14
15
16
17
18

Fig. 129. Arteries of right armpit and shoulder 529 317 919 227:

1 — axillary artery 539 891 319 988

2 — thoraco-acromial artery 981 516 719 312

3 — acromial branch 214 328 712 918

4 — deltoid branch 594 716 018 988

5 — pectoral branch 598 317 918 227

6 — lateral thoracic artery 598 722 918 213

7 — subscapular artery 598 718 419 087

8 — thoracodorsal artery 594 715 319 812

9 — artery circumflexing the scapula 897 314 421 899

10 — anterior artery, enveloping the humerus 599 816 719 817

11 — posterior artery circumflexing the humerus 219 714 819 814

12 — deep brachial artery 317 818 917 918

13 — superior left collateral artery 891 047 089 517

14 — brachial artery 890 319 210 819

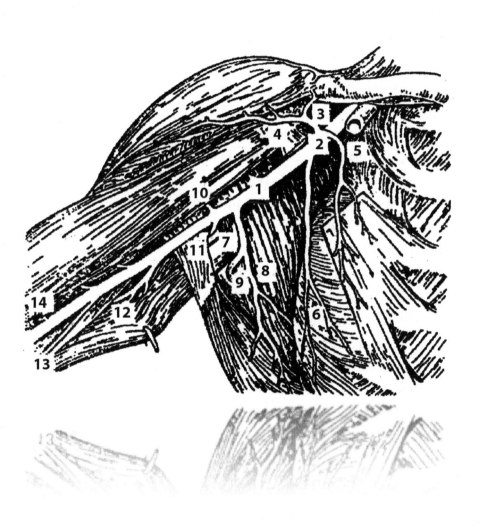

BRANCHES OF THORACIC AORTA 514 712 814 312

BRANCHES OF ABDOMINAL AORTA 548 711 488 211

Fig. 130. Thoracic and abdominal part of aorta 898 121 319 711:

1 — left common carotid artery 898 788 987 128

2 — left subclavian artery 891 061 719 218

3 — internal thoracic artery 598 341 818 941

4 — aortic arch 219 877 549 277

5 — bronchial branches 419 712 819 314

6 — descending part of aorta 519 817 218 217

7 — celiac trunk 594 315 894 715

8 — superior mesenteric artery 398 712 888 422

9 — diaphragm 594 891 794 911

10 — abdominal part of aorta 598 316 488 916

11 — inferior mesentric artery 598 361 988 712

12 — common iliac artery 898 531 314 717

13 — external iliac artery 819 415 919 215

14 — internal iliac artery 584 319 914 899

15 — median sacral artery 598 713 818 213

16 — iliopsoas artery 519 388 918 916

17 — lumbar artery 489 712 319 272

18 — ovarian artery 519 648 319 788

19 — right renal artery 528 316 888 716

20 — inferior diaphragmatic artery 598 318 918 999

21 — intercostal artery 548 316 689 766

22 — ascending aorta 598 712 898 612

23 — brachiocephalic trunk 608 714 318 224

24 — right subclavian artery 598 317 819 227

25 — right common carotid artery 919 421 818 728

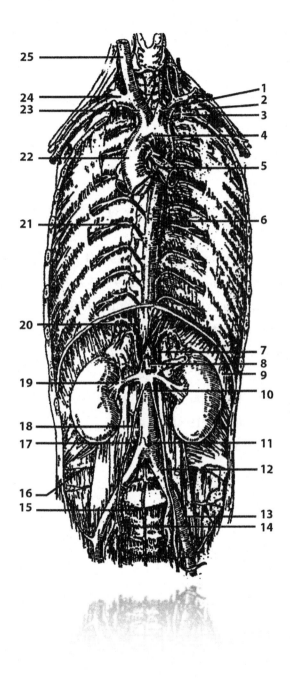

Fig. 131-A Leg arteries 319 421 919 724:

A — Front View:

1 — patellar articular network 219 214 319 814

2 — tendon of tibialis anterior muscle 519 717 919 817

3 — tendon of the long extensor digitorum 319 488 519 318

4 — dorsal artery of foot 514 317 814 217

5 — long extensor of thumb 529 361 819 711

6 — long peroneal muscle 524 782 344 522

7 — long extensor digitorum 598 718 324 201

8 — anterior tibial artery 219 488 714 918

9 — bursa of knee joint 589 412 919 812

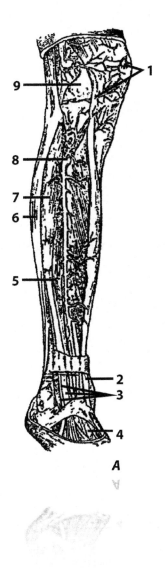

A

Fig. 131-B Leg arteries 319 421 919 724:

B — rear view:

1 — popliteal artery 988 612 818 719

2 — superior lateral knee artery 548 321 748 244

3, 10 — sural artery 549 365 814 775

4 — inferior lateral knee artery 528 312 718 422

5 — posterior tibial recurrent artery 598 711 989 321

6 — anterior tibial artery 569 712 989 212

7 — peroneal artery 594 782 914 882

8 — posterior tibial artery 589 766 914 861

9 — inferior medial knee artery 595 814 315 914

11 — superior medial knee artery 514 317 814 919

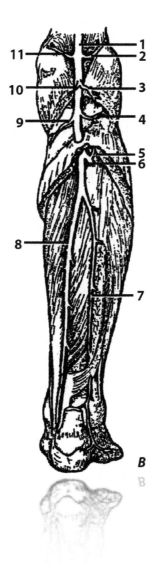

B

VEINS OF SYSTEMIC CIRCULATION 514 312 814 212

CARDIAC VEINS 219 317 919 817

Fig. 132. Veins of heart 891 428 319 298:

1 — left coronary vein 514 816 718 316

2 — posterior vein of left ventricle 429 318 719 888

3 — anterior descending vein 548 712 918 232

4 — posterior interventricular vein 548 716 328 916

5 — anterior vein of right ventricle 548 213 898 263

6 — right margin vein 597 361 326 891

7 — small heart vein 598 712 918 322

8 — coronary sinus 578 916 219 316

9 — oblique vein of left atrium 598 714 319 814

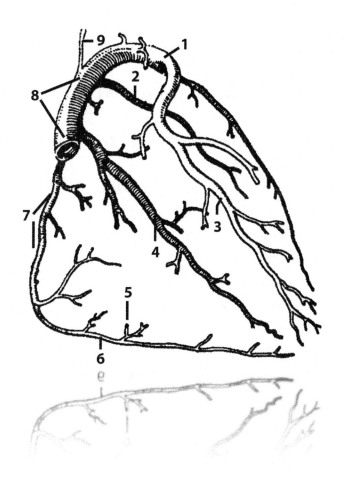

SYSTEM OF SUPERIOR VENA CAVA 898 317 419 217

VEINS OF HEAD AND NECK 598 716 319 816

Fig. 133. Veins of head and face 519 317 919 217:

1 — occipital vein 914 712 298 267

2 — Pterygoid (venous) wreath 591 248 791 260

3 — maxillary vein 598 314 818 914

4 — retromandibular vein 898 314 718 914

5 — internal jugular vein 598 612 719 322

6 — external jugular vein 594 716 814 516

7 — chin vein 598 714 318 914

8 — face vein 599 715 819 316

9 — frontal vein 598 781 428 677

10 — superficial temporal vein 548 327 918 227

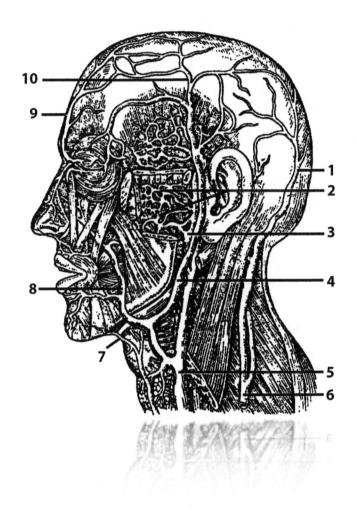

Fig. 134. Vein of thoracic and
abdominal cavities 514 715 914 315:

1 — internal jugular vein 519 317 819 217

2 — external jugular vein 398 601 918 221

3 — subclavian vein 519 371 919 871

4 — brachiocephalic vein 219 378 919 278

5 — upper hollow vein 214 317 814 997

6 — bronchi 519 318 619 228

7 — intercostal vein 549 716 919 226

8 — hemiazygos vein 529 317 818 227

9 — diaphragm 428 713 818 213

10 — beginning of hemiazygos vein 548 712 898 326

11 — inferior hollow vein 549 671 919 871

12 — lumbar vein 589 712 919 261

13 — common iliac vein 548 713 918 781

14 — medial sacral vein 598 717 318 917

15 — internal iliac vein 549 316 814 787

16 — external iliac vein 999 888 719 898

17 — iliopsoas vein 548 791 018 216

18 — square loin muscle 019 321 068 911

19 — the beginning of the azygos 519 217 918 757

20 — azygos vein 729 329 898 888

21 — accessory hemiazygos vein 818 888 068 712

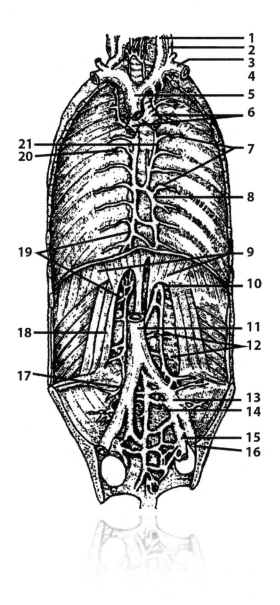

1
2
3
4
5
6
7
8
9
10
11
12
13
14
15
16
17
18
19
20
21

SYSTEM OF INFERIOR VENA CAVA 219 312 819 242

PORTAL VEIN SYSTEM 478 647 319 277

Fig. 135. Portal vein system 478 647 319 277:

1 — superior mesenteric vein 319 841 219 221

2 — stomach 598 718 328 601

3 — left gastroepiploic vein 428 816 968 989

4 — left gastric vein 319 817 298 061

5 — spleen 548 711 918 321

6 — tail of pancreas 549 916 899 716

7 — splenic vein 598 715 328 515

8 — left colic vein 894 312 594 712

9 — descending colon 598 713 818 913

10 — rectum 458 617 918 317

11 — inferior iliac vein 594 316 814 216

12 — medium iliac vein 499 371 819 281

13 — superior iliac vein 519 371 918 991

14 — ileum 548 712 818 912

15 — ascending colon 519 371 819 971

16 — head of pancreas 548 613 718 913

17, 23 — right gastroepiploic vein 519 371 914 881

18 — portal vein 319 817 919 417

19 — cholecystic vein 419 387 918 297

20 — gall bladder 319 214 298 481

21 — duodenum 589 608 488 914

22 — liver 219 712 919 222

24 — pyloric vein 429 716 219 316

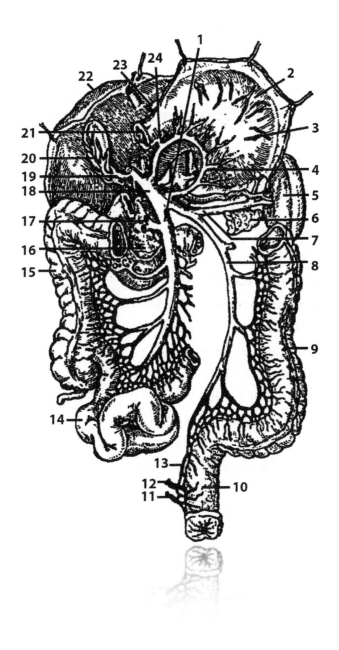

LYMPHATIC SYSTEM 548 716 228 916

Fig. 136. Lymphatic System 519 481 318 881:

1, 2 — parotid lymph minds 519 614 889 714

3 — neck nodes 319 481 519 329

4 — thoracic duct 514 715 914 815

5, 14 — axillary lymph nodes 518 712 818 912

6, 13 — elbow lymph nodes 548 379 918 679

7, 9 — inguinal lymph nodes 214 387 914 297

8 — superficial lymphatic vessels tibia 548 961 558 711

10 — iliac nodes 590 124 397 488

11 — mesenteric nodes 248 718 518 329

12 — chylocyst 519 067 819 297

15 — infraclavicular nodes 598 714 998 294

16 — occipital nodes 319 261 819 811

17 — submandibular nodes 548 312 819 212

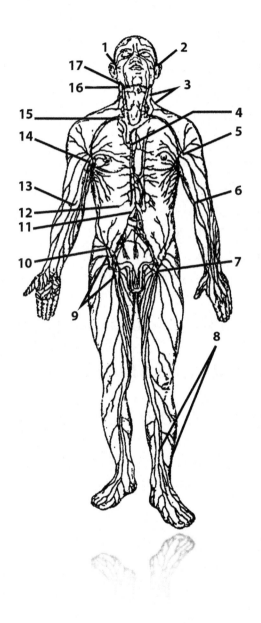

Fig. 137. Structure of lymph nodes 591 148 319 888:

1 — Capsule 519 848 718 949

2 — trabecula 518 716 918 317

3 — crossbar 898 749 219 317

4 — cortex 519 421 319 281

5 — follicles 898 715 984 355

6 — afferent lymphatic vessels 598 741 288 511

7 — medulla 549 378 918 268

8 — efferent lymph vessels 512 789 319 489

9 — Gate of lymph node 598 681 724 918

BLOOD-FORMING ORGANS 498 712 818 292

ORGANS 814 317 914 817

SYSTEMS OF ORGANS 314 815 514 312

ORGANISM AS A WHOLE
419 312 819 212

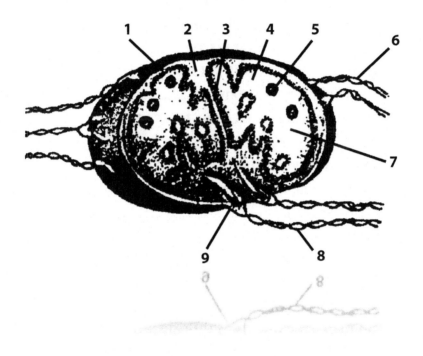

CONTENTS

NOTES

Grigori Grabovoi

Restoration of Matter of Human Being by

Concentrating on Number Sequence

CPSIA information can be obtained at www.ICGtesting.com
Printed in the USA
BVOW11s1223020815

411447BV00016B/389/P